RENAL DIET COOKBOOK

177+ Effective Recipes for Beginners to Pamper and Protect Your Kidneys. Learn how to Avoid Dialysis Danger and Go Back to Sleep Soundly (Satisfying Results in 28 days)

By Dorothy Vandekamp

© Copyright 2020 by Dorothy Vandekamp - All rights reserved.

The content contained within this book may not be reproduced, duplicated, or transmitted without direct written permission from the author or the publisher.

Under no circumstances will any blame or legal responsibility be held against the publisher, or author, for any damages, reparation, or monetary loss due to the information contained within this book. Either directly or indirectly.

Legal Notice:

This book is copyright protected. This book is only for personal use. You cannot amend, distribute, sell, use, quote, or paraphrase any part, or the content within this book, without the consent of the author or publisher.

Disclaimer Notice:

Please note the information contained within this document is for educational and entertainment purposes only. All effort has been executed to present accurate, up-to-date, and reliable, complete information.

No warranties of any kind are declared or implied. Readers acknowledge that the author is not engaging in the rendering of legal, financial, medical, or professional advice. The content within this book has been derived from various sources. Please consult a licensed professional before attempting any techniques outlined in this book.

By reading this document, the reader agrees that under no circumstances is the author responsible for any losses, direct or indirect, which are incurred as a result of the use of the information contained within this document, including, but not limited to, — errors, omissions, or inaccuracies.

TABLE OF CONTENTS

INTRODUCTION **10**
CHAPTER ONE: Understanding Renal Diet **12**
   Causes of acute renal failure 12
   Causes of chronic renal failure 13
   The Role of Sodium in the Body 13
   The Role of Potassium in the Body 14
   The Role of Phosphorus in the Body 15
   Diet for Kidney Failure: What to Eat and What to Avoid 15
   Adapt to Renal Failure 19
CHAPTER TWO: What is Kidney Disease **22**
   Causes of Kidney Disease 23
   Symptoms of Chronic Kidney Failure 23
   Diagnosis for Chronic Kidney Disease 24
   Ultrasound Imaging Diagnosis 25
CHAPTER THREE: 8 Strategic Steps to Control Chronic Kidney Failure **28**
   A Diet for Chronic Kidney Disease 29
CHAPTER FOUR: Kidneys and Low-Carb Diet **33**
CHAPTER FIVE: The Flawless 14-Day Renal Diet Meal Plan **36**
CHAPTER SIX: Breakfast Recipes **44**
   1. Papaya and cranberry jam 44
   2. Lemon curd 45
   3. Poor knight with apple compote 45
   4. Pancakes with raspberries and ricotta 46
   5. Muesli made from rice flakes 47
   6. Muesli mix, low in potassium 47
   7. Bamboo bread (low carb) 48
   8. Open bread with avocado 48
   9. Bircher muesli with papaya 49
   10. Cauliflower and broccoli curry 50
   11. Broccoli and lentil salad with mackerel 50
   12. Broccoli rice gratin (Italian Style) 51

13. Colorful bean salad 52
14. Fennel and Orange Salad 53
15. Fruity egg salad 54
16. Baked mushrooms with pollock cream cheese 55
17. Quinoa oat muesli 55
18. Quark breakfast with mango 56
19. Blueberry Pancakes 57
20. Banana Breakfast Pancakes 58
21. Tuna Spinach Sandwich 59
22. Cranberry Quinoa Salad 60

CHAPTER SEVEN: Poultry and Meat Recipes 63

23. Summer pot pie 63
24. Grilled turkey with lime 64
25. Curry turkey casserole 65
26. Grilled Chicken Salad 66
27. Makhani Chicken 67
28. Moroccan chicken 69
29. Chicken stuffed with herbs and ricotta cheese 70
30. Chicken salad with cranberries and tarragon 71
31. Roast beef meatloaf with protein-free bread 72
32. Pork loin with herbs 73
33. Zucchini cream with chicken 74
34. Beef carpaccio 75
35. Low-protein fusilli with meat sauce 76
36. Ginger Chicken 76
37. Beef stew with rice 77

CHAPTER EIGHT: Lunch Recipes 80

38. Chick Curry (Thai Chicken) 80
39. Fried breaded lasagna with marinara sauce 81
40. Baked Mushrooms with Pumpkin and Chipotle Polenta 82
41. Quinoa salad with chickpeas and feta 83
42. White Bean Salad 84
43. Omelette and summer vegetables 85
44. Elderberry asparagus with herbal cream cheese 85

45. Soup of green asparagus 86
46. Potato salad with asparagus 87
47. Chicken and asparagus salad with watercress.. 88
48. Chicken and zucchini salad with nuts 89
49. Veal kidneys 90
50. Zucchini risotto with kidneys 91
51. Protein-free bucatini with broccoli... 92
52. Protein-free spaghetti carbonara 93
53. Asparagus in salad with poached eggs 94
54. Protein-free bread dumplings... 95
55. Protein-free tagliatelle with courgettes and pistachios............................. 96
56. Protein-free rice salad with Mediterranean pesto..................................... 97
57. Protein-free Margherita pizza... 98
58. Protein-free spaghetti "alla Norma".. 99
59. Protein-free penne with tuna and basil 100
60. Omelette with onions 100
61. Lentils with cotechino 101
62. Pizzoccheri 103
63. Butterflies with hake fillets and courgette flowers.................................. 104
64. Pasta and chickpeas.. 105
65. Pasta with sardines 107
66. Rice with baby octopus and radicchio 108

CHAPTER NINE: Soup and Stew Recipes 111
67. Chili con carne 111
68. Creamy chicken soup with wild rice and asparagus................................ 111
69. Cold cucumber soup... 112
70. Pumpkin and walnut puree 113
71. Andean soup... 114
72. Bean and pepper soup with coriander 115
73. Bean and ham soup with bread 116
74. Hearty vegetable soup with bacon 117
75. Mexican-style chicken and vegetable soup 118
76. Mexican bean soup 119
77. Bean and potato stew... 120

78. Clear soup with vegetables 121

79. Bean stew with beef fillet 122

80. Nutmeg pumpkin soup with kidney beans 123

81. Zucchini soup 123

82. Quick pea soup 124

83. Tomato soup made from fresh tomatoes 125

84. Chickpea soup with croutons 126

85. Chestnut and chickpea soup 127

CHAPTER TEN: Salads 130

86. Hawaiian Chicken Salad 130

87. Grated carrot salad with lemon-Dijon vinaigrette 130

88. Tuna macaroni salad 131

89. Couscous salad 131

90. Fruity zucchini salad 132

91. Cucumber salad, pulled through slowly 133

92. Tortellini salad 133

93. Farmer's Salad 134

94. Orange and grapefruit salad with date stripes 135

95. Chicken and asparagus salad with watercress 135

96. Buckwheat salad 137

97. Salad with feta and taggiasca olives 138

98. Kartoffelsalat 140

CHAPTER ELEVEN: Vegetarian Recipes 143

99. Spring vegetables with tofu from the wok 143

100. Asparagus and carrot salad with burrata 144

101. Quinoa Salad Winning 144

102. Spinach Mango Vegetables 145

103. Braised Swiss chard with garlic and balsamic vinegar 146

104. Snow peas all with thyme 147

105. Cauliflower and fresh dill 147

106. Zucchini and corn stir-fry 148

107. Marinated zucchini 148

108. "Cooked water" 150

CHAPTER TWELVE: Desserts and Sweets 153

109. Oatmeal and berry muffins 153
110. Crunchy Blueberry and Apples 154
111. Raspberry feast meringue with cream diplomat 155
112. Pear crumble with vanilla sauce 156
113. Rice casserole with cherries 156
114. Crepes with protein-free flour 157
115. Wine biscuits with protein-free flour 158
116. Strawberry tiramisu 159
117. Donut-shaped cake with white icing and coloured sprinkles 160
118. Amarena dessert 162
119. Peach ice cream 162
120. Fruit rice 163
121. Tiramisu 163
122. Fake berry cheesecake 164
123. Bread cake 165
124. Walnut and hazelnut cake 167
125. Sandy cake 168
126. Pineapple cake 168
127. Lemon cake 169
128. Very soft cake 170

CHAPTER THIRTEEN: Snacks, Entrées and Sides 173

129. Pear crumble with vanilla sauce 173
130. Rice casserole with cherries 173
131. Tantalizing artichokes 174
132. Sweet and sour onions 175
133. Carrot salad 176
134. Tofu patties 176
135. Potato gratin 177
136. Cucumber salad, pulled through slowly 177
137. Turnip vegetables 178
138. Cucumber salad with mint 179
139. Green beans in salad 179
140. Stewed lettuce 180
141. Gratin onions 181

142. Zucchini with protein-free bechamel 181
143. Friselle with cherry tomatoes 182
144. Crispy polenta 183
145. "Frattau" bread 184

CHAPTER FOURTEEN: Spreads, Dips, Appetizers and Sauces 187

146. Salmon Cream Cheese 187
147. Spicy spread 187
148. Bulgur spread 188
149. Apple and onion lard 188
150. Zucchini spread 189
151. Vegetable spread 189
152. Herbal Cupcakes 190
153. Salmon cream cheese 191
154. Cold cucumber soup 191
155. Thick cream of carrots (Crecy potage) with protein-free croutons 192
156. Pumpkin cream with prawns and quinoa 193
157. Provençal pie with low-protein artichokes 194
158. Gratin Scallops 195
159. Red onion tart with protein-free flour 196
160. Carrot flans with green sauce 198

CHAPTER FIFTEEN: Fish and Seafood Recipes 201

161. Rissole of dried codfish or codfish pancakes 201
162. Steamed Jamaican Fish 201
163. Shrimp and apple stir-fry 202
164. Spicy shrimp linguine 203
165. Spaghetti with shrimps 204
166. Protein-free spaghetti with clams 205
167. Salmon with horseradish cream 206
168. Sole rolls 207
169. Swordfish rolls with mango sauce 209
170. White mussel soup 211

CHAPTER SIXTEEN: Smoothies, Juices and Beverages 213

171. Seasonal berry drinks 213
172. Fresh Lemonade 214

173. Blueberry Shake 214
CHAPTER SEVENTEEN: Low-Protein Desserts 216
174. Low-Protein Apple Pie 216
175. Low-Protein Carrot Cake 217
176. Low-Protein Apple Strudel 218
177. Low-Protein Panna Cotta with Strawberries and Raspberries 219
178. Low-Protein Tart with Citrus Jam 221
CONCLUSION 224
Composition of Some Types of Vegetables and Fruits 224
What the Numbers Associated with the Most Common Diets Want to Say 225
A Practical Strategy to Reduce the Potassium Content in Vegetables 226

INTRODUCTION

Chronic CKD is a major public health problem. A systematic review, based on population studies from developed countries, described an average prevalence of 7.2% (individuals over age 30). According to data from the EPIRCE study, it affects approximately 10% of the Spanish adult population and more than 20% of those over 60 years of age, and it is also undiagnosed. In patients with diseases as frequent as arterial hypertension (AHT) or diabetes mellitus (DM), the prevalence of CKD can be 35-40%. The magnitude of the problem is even greater given the increase in kidney-related morbidity and mortality, especially cardiovascular.

CKD is considered the final common destination for a constellation of pathologies that affect the kidney chronically and irreversibly. Once the diagnostic and therapeutic measures of primary kidney disease have been exhausted, CKD involves common and generally independent protocols for action.

The most frequent causes of ERCA with their corresponding links are described in this eBook. Often more than one cause coexists and enhances kidney damage.

- Diabetic nephropathy
- Arteriosclerotic vascular disease, nephroangiosclerosis, ischemic nephropathy. Concepts all that have in common the presence of arterial hypertension.
- Primary or secondary glomerular disease to systemic disease
- Congenital and hereditary nephropathies
- Interstitial nephropathies
- Prolonged obstruction of the urinary tract (including lithiasis)
- Urinary tract infections
- Systemic diseases (lupus, vasculitis, myeloma ....)

In this chapter, we will review the clinical aspects and conservative management of CKD. Diagnoses and treatments of specific renal diseases are discussed in the corresponding chapters. And nutrition needed to canter the diseases with different recipes.

CHAPTER ONE: Understanding Renal Diet

4 to 6 litters of blood circulate in the body, depending on the weight of the body. Blood is transported through the renal arteries to the kidneys. Around 1,500 litres of blood pass through the kidneys every day, which are cleansed by the work of around a million nephrons.

Nephrons consist of small filters that separate water, salts, and impurities from the blood, called glomeruli. In it, protein and blood cells remain. Small channels transport the filtered fluid (primary urine). There are cells of a specific type (tubular cells) that cause the blood to return to water and salts such as sodium, calcium, phosphorus, and magnesium. The remainder of the fluid is discharged as final urine.

Blood pressure and the concentration of certain hormones that affect the functioning of these cells depend on the amount of salt absorbed by the tubular cells. Thus, the kidneys regulate the water and salt balance in the body. Conversely, the kidneys also affect blood pressure (for example, more water and sodium are secreted into it when blood pressure drops).

Kidney damage can occur both suddenly and as a result of the process of long-term illness. Acute renal failure (ONN), characterized by a rapid increase in keratinizing and a decrease in diuresis, and even complete anuria, often requiring renal replacement therapy, develops when the kidneys are exposed to a damaging factor for a short period. This disorder can develop within a few hours to 7 days.

Nonetheless, acute failure can lead to full recovery within a few months, and it depends primarily on the type of primary illness. However, if the kidney is gradually damaged during the long disease process (lasting at least three months), the most serious forms of chronic kidney disease develop severe chronic kidney failure and end-stage renal disease requiring dialysis.

The conditions of impaired blood flow, particular and non-specific inflammation and immunological factors and substances toxic to the kidneys are among the factors that impair kidney function; all processes can impair urinary tract patentability and chronic diseases such as diabetes and hypertension.

Causes of acute renal failure

The factors responsible for acute kidney damage are divided into so-called perennial, renal, and renal. The first, most common category includes conditions that disturb kidney blood flow, including:

- decreased circulating the blood volume due to haemorrhage, dehydration, excessive diuresis, seepage into the body cavities, or extensive burns and injuries;
- heart disease characterized by a sudden decrease in stroke volume;

- states of the sudden increase in the volume of the vascular bed due to a vascular tone disorder (sepsis, antihypertensive, electrolyte disturbances, cirrhosis);
- autoregulation of renal blood flow due to the use of non-steroidal anti-inflammatory drugs, cyclooxygenase inhibitors, or angiotensin receptor blockers (drugs used in hypertension);
- conditions of excessive blood viscosity, including hematologic malignancies
- obstruction of the vessels supplying the kidneys due to a blood clot, embolism, aneurysm, external pressure, e.g., by a tumour or inflammation.

Renal factors that damage organ parenchyma include all glomerular inflammatory processes (autoimmune, allergic, viral, bacterial, idiopathic), systemic vacuities, thrombotic microangiopathy, cholesterol embolism, malignant hypertension, autoimmune diseases including systemic lupus erythematosus and scleroderma systemic, damage to the renal parenchyma due to prolonged impaired blood supply, toxins - including contrast agents and drugs (including cyclosporine, cisplatin, some antibiotics, captopril, methotrexate, indinavir, acyclovir, ethylene glycol and methanol and - attention - popular non-steroidal drugs anti-inflammatory), as well as cancerous infiltrates.

Last but not least, the causes of ONN are conditions that obstruct the urinary tract (also within the bladder) by urolithiasis, blood clots, fragments of damaged nipples, external pressure, e.g. by a cancerous tumour or in diseases of the prostate in men, interruption of the urinary tract or damage to the urethra.

Causes of chronic renal failure

In contrast to ONN, in this disease entity kidney damage occurs gradually, primarily in the course of chronic diseases, such as:

- diabetes mellitus (diabetic nephropathy),
- hypertension (hypertensive nephropathy),
- glomerulonephritis and tubulointerstitial inflammatory processes,
- polycystic degeneration,
- systemic diseases, including sarcoidosis and amyloidosis
- less often long-term impaired blood flow or outflow of urine,
- plasma myeloma,
- HIV nephropathy
- Genetically determined syndromes, e.g., Alport syndrome.

The Role of Sodium in the Body

Sodium is one of the elements necessary for the proper functioning of the body. He is primarily responsible for water and electrolyte management, but also has other functions. What are his other roles? Are there serious effects of sodium excess and deficiency? How to introduce a diet that will allow us to reduce sodium intake?

Sodium has important functions in the body, and disturbances in its concentration can cause serious problems. The main tasks of this valuable element include:

- maintaining the osmotic balance of the body in the extracellular fluids of the body - this means that it regulates the volume of water in the body and protects us from dehydration,
- maintaining acid-base balance (together with potassium and chlorine),
- involved in the conduction of nerve impulses - sodium is a potassium antagonist, and this element creates a concentration difference on both sides of the cell membrane, thus enabling the transmission of impulses. This process is responsible for the state of smooth muscle, skeletal and heart tension,
- participation in the process of glucose and amino acid transport across cell membranes,
- activating salivary amylase - a digestive enzyme present in saliva.

Normal sodium concentration in the body is 135-145 mmol /l, and its maintenance is responsible for the renin-angiotensin-aldosterone system. It is a complex hormonal - enzyme system that also regulates the volume of water in the body.

The Role of Potassium in the Body

Potassium belongs to microelements and has many essential functions. Potassium allows our cells to transmit electrical impulses, but potassium also helps maintain adequate blood pressure and muscle tone.

Potassium is therefore an electrolyte, controlling muscle function. It allows the generation of electrical impulses in our body's cells, including heart muscle cells, i.e. it is responsible for each heartbeat. Potassium plays the same skeletal muscle function.

Potassium is a sodium antagonist and its opposite action includes reducing the volume of extracellular fluids, which helps control the amount of water in the body. This role of potassium also can maintain healthy blood pressure by lowering it.

Potassium is involved in processes where our cells synthesize proteins, which are muscle building blocks. Potassium is one of the factors controlling muscle building and helping maintain healthy muscle mass.

Potassium, also a calcium antagonist, is responsible for proper muscle tone (so-called tonus) by elevating its tone.

Potassium also helps maintain acid-base balance, thus maintaining the body's homeostasis.

If our body functions properly, the potassium-sodium balance is maintained. Disorders in these microelement concentrations cause one of the most common and severe civilization diseases, i.e., hypertension and heart disease. Low potassium levels promote these diseases, unlike sodium.

People rarely have potassium deficiency or bearing. However, this happens when our body's functioning is disturbed.

Potassium deficiency, or hypokalaemia, may occur when using high blood pressure diuretics, for prolonged vomiting or diarrhoea, and with some kidney problems. Hypokalaemia symptoms are weak, flaccid muscles, arrhythmias, and slightly increased blood pressure.

Hyperkalaemia, too high in potassium, causes dangerous arrhythmia. Hyperkalaemia occurs when kidneys are weak, infections are severe, and heart medicines are taken.

The Role of Phosphorus in the Body

Because up to 85% of phosphorus is found in bones and teeth, its proper structure must be maintained. It also occurs in soft and cell membranes, i.e., muscle, heart, and brain tissues. Also plays an essential role in growing and reconstructing or repairing damaged tissues. As one of the elements involved in human body processes, phosphorus is also an energy transmitter. These minerals convert food into energy that translates into muscle work.

Phosphorus also ensures proper nerve and brain function and is involved in many chemical reactions and metabolic processes in our body. Maintains overall body vitality. It also plays an important role in heart work. For researchers, it is an important carrier of genetic information because it is a DNA component.

Diet for Kidney Failure: What to Eat and What to Avoid

In the renal failure diet, some nutrient intake such as sodium, phosphorus, potassium, and protein must be controlled. In the most severe cases where kidneys no longer function well or dialysis, it is also necessary to control the number of fluids ingested daily. Includes water, juices, and soups.

When talking about kidney failure, it means that the ability of the kidneys to filter waste from the blood and form urine is diminished, causing specific residues and minerals, such as those mentioned above, to accumulate in the blood and can cause serious consequences, due to the restriction of these nutrients in the diet.

These individuals need to reduce protein intake such as meats, fish, grains, and some types of fruits and legumes such as orange and kiwi. However, for potassium-rich foods, some techniques can be used to reduce the amount of potassium in fruits and vegetables, such as peeling them before eating them.

Foods to be controlled

Renal insufficiency can be acute or chronic, so food restrictions in the diet vary according to the type of inadequacy and the stage in which the disease is found.

Ideally, in these situations, the individual should go to a nutritionist specialized in the area to develop an individual nutritional plan based on the laboratory tests of the person, so the foods mentioned below should be consumed in moderation, since that the fact that they are ingested or not will depend on laboratory values:

Foods high in potassium

The kidneys of people with renal insufficiency have difficulty removing excess potassium from the blood, so those people need to control the intake of this mineral by avoiding abuse of them.

Potassium-rich foods are:

- Fruits: avocado, banana, coconut, fig, guava, kiwi, orange, papaya, passion fruit, tangerine, grape, raisins, plums, prune, melon, apricot, blackberries, dates;
- Vegetables: potato, sweet potato, cassava, Creole celery, carrot, chard, beet, celery, cabbage, Brussel sprouts, radish, tomatoes, canned palm, spinach, turnip, and chicory;
- Legumes: beans, lentils, corn, peas, chickpea, soybeans, beans;
- Whole grains: wheat, rice, oats;
- Whole foods: biscuits, whole wheat pasta, breakfast cereals;
- Oleaginous: peanut, cashew, almonds, hazelnuts;
- Industrialized products: chocolate, tomato sauce, meat, and chicken broth tablets;
- Drinks: coconut water, sports drinks, black tea, green tea, matte tea;
- Seeds: sesame, flaxseed;
- Paper or sugar cane guarapo;
- Salt light

Too much potassium can cause muscle weakness, arrhythmias, and cardiac arrest, so the diet for chronic renal failure has to be individualized and accompanied by

the doctor and the nutritionist, who will evaluate the appropriate amounts of nutrients that each person should ingest.

How to reduce potassium in the food

Some strategies can help reduce the amount of potassium in fruits and vegetables; these are:

- Peel fruits and vegetables;
- Cut and rinse food thoroughly;

- Place the plants to soak in water in the refrigerator for a day, before use;
- Place the food in a pot with water and boil for 10 minutes. Then drain the water and cook again with water and then prepare the food as desired.

Another important suggestion is to avoid the use of pressure cookers and microwaves to prepare meals since these techniques concentrate the potassium content in food by not allowing water to be changed.

Foods rich in phosphorus

Phosphorus-rich foods should also be consumed moderately by people with chronic renal failure to control kidney function. These foods are:

- Canned sins;
- Salted, smoked, and sausage meats such as sausages and sausages;
- Bacon, bacon;
- Yolk;
- Milk and derivatives;
- Soy and derivatives;
- Beans, lentils, peas, corn;
- Oilseeds such as cashew, almonds, and peanuts;
- Seeds such as sesame and flaxseed;
- Coconut sweet;
- Beer, cola, and hot chocolate.

Symptoms of excess phosphorus are itchy body, hypertension, and mental confusion, and people with kidney failure should keep an eye on these signs.

Protein-rich foods

People with chronic renal failure need to control the consumption of proteins because, during their metabolism, toxic wastes are produced that accumulate in the blood, and cannot be eliminated. This is why it is essential to avoid excessive consumption of meat, fish, eggs, milk, and derivatives since they are foods rich in protein.

Ideally, a person with kidney failure should eat one small beef steak at lunch and dinner and one glass of milk or yogurt per day. However, this amount varies according to how the kidney function is, being more restrictive in those people in whom the kidney almost does not work.

Foods rich in salt and water

People with kidney failure also need to control salt intake, since the excess increases blood pressure and forces the kidney to work, further impairing the function of this organ. The same happens with the excess of liquids since these people produce little urine, and the excess of liquids ends up accumulating in the organism, causing problems such as swelling and dizziness.

Therefore, the use of:

- Salt;
- Sauces such as ketchup, mayonnaise, aioli, among others;
- Tomato paste;
- Condiments such as cubes, soy sauce, and Worcestershire sauce;
- Canned food and frozen prepared food;
- Snacks, chips, and crackers with salt;
- Fast food;
- Powdered or canned soups.

To avoid excess salt, a good option is to use aromatic herbs to season foods such as parsley, garlic, and basil. The doctor or nutritionist will indicate the appropriate amount of salt and water allowed for each person individually.

How to choose snacks

Restrictions on the feeding of the renal patient can make it difficult to choose snacks. Therefore, the 3 most important recommendations for choosing healthy snacks are:

- Eat always cooked fruit (cook twice), never reusing cooking water, and it must be discarded;
- Restrict industrialized and processed foods that are generally rich in salt or sugars, preferring homemade preparations;
- Avoid the intake of protein foods in snacks.

Diet for acute renal failure

The diet for acute renal failure is usually performed at the hospital level, because it is a situation that occurs suddenly and is treated in the hospital, being carefully calculated by the nutritionist, and may even be necessary to use food through a route intravenously to administer the number of nutrients that the individual requires.

In general, renal function is usually restored, and the individual receives specific instructions on what they can eat to avoid the accumulation of toxins that are eliminated through the kidneys. Normally this diet is usually low in protein, potassium, salt, and phosphorus, as in chronic renal failure, until the function of the kidneys completely returns to normal.

Adapt to Renal Failure

Discovering that you have kidney failure can be a shock, even if you have known for a long time that your kidneys are not working well. But starting dialysis treatment doesn't have to say that the ones you enjoy are over. It may take a little time to adapt to your new routine, but you are not alone. Your doctors, nurses, and social workers can help you.

Depression and anxiety

Depression is a feeling of sadness that extends for a long time. Anxiety is a feeling of nervousness that comes and goes.

It is normal for you to be nervous when you are going through significant changes in your life, mainly if these changes affect your health and well-being. When you start dialysis treatment, you may have to change your daily routine, your diet, and the type of activities you do. You will probably experience different feelings as you get used to this new lifestyle, such as sadness, fear, regret, and anger. You may not immediately understand what you are feeling, but you may notice that you feel strange.

Symptoms of depression are:

- Changes in sleeping patterns (sleeping too much or having trouble sleeping)
- Loss of interest in those activities you used to enjoy
- Loss of appetite

Some symptoms of anxiety are:

- Heart Rate Acceleration
- Sweating
- breathe too fast
- difficulty thinking about anything except what worries you

You must know that you are not alone. Most people have gone through what you are going through. Many people have felt like you. It is also essential that you know that you do not have to live with these feelings. Help is available. Talk to your social worker about the different ways to start feeling better. You may also find support groups useful.

Exercise

Exercise is a great way to improve your health. Most people, though undergoing dialysis treatment, can and should exercise.

People who regularly exercise feel better physically and emotionally. Exercise benefits include:

- Mood improvement
- Improvement of heart and lung health

- Weightless
- Joint pain reduction
- Greater flexibility

Exercise does not have to be difficult or painful. If it hurts to perform a certain exercise, you shouldn't do it! There are many ways to exercise without experiencing pain or discomfort. Consider practicing low impact exercises.

These are exercises that do not cause too much tension in the joints. Some examples of low impact exercises are:

- Hike
- Swimming
- riding a bicycle
- Yoga
- Pilates
- Use of elliptical machine
- Tai Chi
- Stretching
- Climbing stairs

You can walk in your neighbourhood or the mall. Or you can practice yoga at home on the floor of your living room. Your doctor can help you design an exercise plan that is safe for you, and that suits your dialysis itinerary.

Job

You may be able to continue working during your dialysis treatment. Working can help you feel happier and fulfilled. If you have health insurance through your work, staying in it will help you keep your insurance.

If you want or need to continue working during your dialysis treatment, talk to your doctor about your treatment options. Certain types of dialysis allow you to keep a more flexible schedule during the day.

For example, if you choose night haemodialysis (at night), in the centre or at home, you can perform your dialysis treatments at night, while you sleep. This is also possible with cyclist assisted continuous peritoneal dialysis (CCPD).

If you decide to continue working during your dialysis treatment, you must know your limits. You may feel tired or weak throughout the day. If you receive peritoneal dialysis treatment and make your exchanges, you must have a clean place in your work to do the exchanges. If you receive haemodialysis treatment, you should not lift heavy objects or put pressure on the arm of your vascular access.

CHAPTER TWO: What is Kidney Disease

Chronic renal failure or uremia is the inability of the kidneys to produce or produce low-quality urine ("like water") because sufficient toxic waste has not been removed. Although some patients continue to urinate, it is not possible for most. The significant thing, however, is not the quantity, but the urine composition or quality.

The kidneys are two "bean-shaped" organs, located at the sides of the spine in the dorsal wall of the body. They are brown, each weighing about 150 grams, about 12 centimeters in length, 6 centimeters in width, and 3 centimeters in thickness. Each kidney has an endocrine gland attached to it (it produces vital substances within the body) in the upper part, called the adrenal gland.

The "purifiers" where the blood is filtered and cleaned are the kidneys. They generate urine containing water, toxins, and salts that have been collected throughout the body by the blood, and that must be eliminated. Other activities, such as reproduction, also involve them because they make sex hormones; regulate the amount of phosphorus and calcium in the bones; regulate the tension in the blood vessels; and produce substances involved in blood clotting.

When only 5 percent of the total kidney or nephron philters work, renal insufficiency appears. The basic unit of the kidney is the nephron, about 1 million of which are found in each organ. Each nephron is formed by a component, the glomerulus, and a transport system, the tubule, that acts as a filter.

The glomerulus philters some of the blood that reaches the kidneys and passes through the tubules, where different processes of excretion and reabsorption occur that give rise to the urine that is eventually removed.

Renal blood flow (RBF, or the amount of blood that reaches the kidney per minute) is about 1.1 liters per minute for adults. Of the 0.6 plasma liters that enter through the arterioles into the glomerulus, 20 percent are filtered, an operation called renal glomerular filtration.

Therefore, the volume of plasma filtered by the kidneys per unit of time is the renal glomerular filtrate. Per day, the quantity of filtered plasma is 135 to 160 liters. Between 98 percent and 99 percent of the renal glomerular filtration rate is reabsorbed by the tubules to prevent fluid loss, resulting in urine removal of between one and two liters per day.

It means that one or more of the renal functions are altered when a kidney disorder happens. However, not all functions are altered in the same proportion; if, for example, two-thirds of the nephrons cease to function, significant changes may not occur because the remaining nephrons adapt; changes in hormonal production may also go unnoticed, and then the only way to detect a decrease in the number of nephrons that continue to function is to calculate renal glomerular filtration.

Causes of Kidney Disease

Diseases and conditions that usually cause chronic kidney disease include:

- Type 1 and 2 Diabetes
- Hypertension
- Glomerulonephritis, which is inflammation of the glomeruli, functional units of the kidneys where blood filtration occurs
- Interstitial Nephritis
- Polycystic Kidney Disease and Other Congenital Diseases That Affect Kidneys
- Prolonged urinary tract obstruction due to specific conditions such as prostatic hyperplasia, kidney stones, and some cancers
- Vesicoureteral reflux
- Recurrent renal infection also called pyelonephritis
- Autoimmune Diseases
- Kidney injury or trauma
- Overuse of painkillers and other medicines
- Use of some toxic chemicals
- Kidney Artery Problems
- Reflux Nephropathy

Chronic renal failure leads to an accumulation of fluid and waste in the body. This disease affects most body systems and functions, including red blood cell production, blood pressure control, vitamin D levels, and bone health.

Risk factors

- Diabetes
- Hypertension
- Heart diseases
- Smoke
- Obesity
- High cholesterol
- Be African American, Native American, or Asian American
- Have a family history of kidney disease
- 65 years or older

Symptoms of Chronic Kidney Failure

Early symptoms of chronic renal failure usually also frequently occur in other diseases, and maybe the only signs of renal failure until it is advanced.

Symptoms may include:

- General malaise and fatigue
- Generalized itching (itching) and dry skin
- Headaches
- Unintentional Weight Loss
- Loss of appetite
- Nausea

Other symptoms that may appear, especially when kidney function worsens include:

- Abnormally light or dark skin
- Bone pain
- Drowsiness and confusion
- Difficulty concentrating and reasoning
- Numbness in hands, feet, and other body areas
- Muscle spasms or cramps
- Bad breath
- Easy bruising, bleeding, or bloody stools
- Excessive thirst
- Frequent hiccups
- Low level of sexual interest and impotence
- Interruption of the menstrual period (amenorrhea)
- Sleep disorders such as insomnia, restless legs syndrome, and sleep apnoea
- Swelling of hands and legs (edema)
- Vomiting, usually in the morning.

Diagnosis for Chronic Kidney Disease

The general precepts of the practice of internal medicine should be applied. The diagnosis of acute renal failure and its differential criteria are addressed in the corresponding section.

Clinic history

Particular attention should be given to urinary symptoms such as nocturnal, polyuria, polydipsia, dysuria, or haematuria. A complete history of systemic diseases, exposure to renal toxins, infections, and possible family history of kidney disease must also be obtained.

Physical exploration

Weight, height, and possible malformations and developmental disorders should be recorded. It is important to take blood pressure, the examination of the fundus, examination of the cardiovascular system and chest, and abdominal palpation looking for palpable masses or kidneys with lumbar contact. In men, a rectal examination is essential to examine the prostate. Signs of edema can be seen on the extremities, and the state of peripheral pulses must be explored.

Biochemical parameters

Urinalysis: haematuria, proteinuria, cylinders (blood cylinders), evaluation of renal function. Alterations associated with CKD: anemia, mineral metabolism (Ca, P, and PTH), acid-base balance.

Ultrasound Imaging Diagnosis

Mandatory tests in all cases to first verify that there are two kidneys, measure their size, analyse their morphology, and rule out urinary obstruction.

Small kidneys (below 9 cm, depending on the body surface) indicate chronicity and irreversibility. Normal-sized kidneys favour the diagnosis of an acute process. However, polycystic kidney disease, amyloidosis, or diabetes can occur with healthy or enlarged kidneys.

If the kidneys have a size difference greater than 2 cm, this may be due to pathology of the renal artery, vesicoureteral reflux, or varying degrees of unilateral renal hypoplasia.

Eco-Doppler

It is the first renal imaging scan in any patient. Inexperienced hands are the first diagnostic step of unit or bilateral renal artery stenosis.

Duplex Doppler: It has the advantage of providing anatomical and functional data of the renal arteries. Direct visualization of the renal artery (mode B) is combined with the measurement (Doppler) of blood flow and its characteristics.

Intravenous urography

Not indicated for the diagnosis of CKD, since the information it provides is limited because no contrast is eliminated, this being also nephrotoxic, being able to precipitate the entry into dialysis. It has been falling into disuse with ultrasound benefits.

Digital angiography

The gold standard for the diagnosis of renal vascular diseases is arteriography, but it has the disadvantage of contrast toxicity.

The first examination at this time in any patient is the performance of a doppler, and later if the renal function is normal, a CT angiography or a magnetic antiresonance can be indicated, according to the experience of each centre.

Angio-CT or helical Scanner: Its most significant advantage is the administration of intravenous contrast, which allows visualizing the calibre of the light and the characteristics of the arterial wall in three dimensions. Its limitation is contrast toxicity in a patient with renal impairment.

Magnetic antiresonance: It is an increasingly used technique in patients with normal renal function and not recommended in patients with grade 3-4 renal insufficiency, given the gadolinium toxicity (See Nephrogenic systemic fibrosis).

Angiography with CO_2 obviates contrast toxicity, but the risk of aeroembolism disease in patients with peripheral artery disease must be kept in mind.

Modern techniques of antiresonance with image intensification offer excellent information about the vascular tree without using gadolinium.

Renal biopsy

It is an invasive and risk-free procedure, indicated when there are diagnostic doubts of primary kidney disease or the degree of chronicity of tissue damage. We must assess their possible risks against the potential benefits of the information you can provide. If it is done in the early stages of the ERC, your information may be useful. In advanced stages, we will often encounter sclerosed and terminal kidneys.

CHAPTER THREE: 8 Strategic Steps to Control Chronic Kidney Failure

(1) Seek treatment for hypertension

The pressure is now considered the leading cause of chronic renal failure. According to nephrologist Nestor Schor, professor at Unifesp, the increase in blood pressure damages the blood vessels of the kidneys and may cause hypertensive nephropathy. "This way, the organ becomes overloaded, and little by little loses its filtering capacity," he explains. Taking care of hypertension is essential even when it is not the cause of chronic renal failure, as it becomes even more important in the advanced stage of the disease.

(2) Control of diabetes

"Diabetes is the second leading cause of chronic renal failure," says nephrologist Lucio Roberto Requião Moura of Hospital Israelita Albert Einstein. This is because the disease triggers the so-called diabetic nephropathy, a change in kidney vessels that leads to a protein loss in the urine. Besides, diabetes favours atherosclerosis, the formation of plaque fat in the arteries that hinders the filtration work of the kidneys. Over time, more and more toxic substances are trapped in the body, which can lead to death. One way to detect the problem, therefore, is to do urine tests to find out if the protein is being eliminated. Those already diagnosed with diabetes need to be more aware of their kidney health.

(3) Watch the weight

Overweight people (Discover their ideal weight) have a higher risk of developing hypertension and diabetes, which is reason enough not to let the scale hand rise, says nephrologist Lucio. Added to this is the fact that obesity alters the way blood reaches the kidneys by the influence of certain hormones, overloading the organ. More so, being overweight is a risk factor for high cholesterol and triglycerides.

(4) Adapt your diet

When it comes to food, analysing the underlying disease that triggered kidney failure is critical. If it is diabetes, for example, the diet should be the right diet for those with diabetes. If it is hypertension, then there should be reduced salt intake. "However, in general, it is recommended that the patient avoid excessive protein intake, especially of animal origin, which gives rise to toxic elements in the body that would make the kidneys work harder," explains nephrologist Nestor. In specific cases of insufficiency yet, there may be retention of potassium in the body. Patients with this problem need to prepare food in a way that causes them to release some of this nutrient. Vegetables, for example, need to be cooked.

(5) Inquire about medications

Self-medication is dangerous even for healthy people. For those with kidney failure, however, use without proper medical evaluation can accelerate kidney deterioration. "The most dangerous are non-hormonal anti-inflammatory drugs," warns nephrologist Lucio. Therefore, explain your problem at the beginning of every medical appointment to avoid aggravating the disease.

(6) Way to drink alcohol

Although no studies are proving the isolated relationship between alcohol intake and chronic renal failure, alcohol abuse compromises the functioning of the body as a whole. Thus, it is recommended to handle consumption. If you are having a drink, however, nephrologist Nestor advises opting for wine. "It contains antioxidants that can help eliminate concentrated toxins in the body.

(7) Put out the cigarette

"Cigarettes are responsible for worsening blood pressure levels and are still involved with hormonal changes that worsen kidney function," explains nephrologist Lucio. Also, smoking triggers a vasoconstriction effect, decreasing the volume of blood filtered by the kidneys. In this case, there is no moderation option. The patient must end the addiction.

(8) Practice exercises

The last recommended care for chronic kidney failure sufferers is regular exercise. "It prevents diabetes, hypertension, obesity, among other problems, and improves circulation and kidney function," says nephrologist Nestor. According to him, any activity is already better than physical inactivity. Still, it is always recommended to seek training that pleases the patient so that he does not feel discouraged over time.

A Diet for Chronic Kidney Disease

Chronic kidney disease (CKD) refers to the continuous deterioration of the kidneys that progress over time (can learn more about the relationship between IRC CKD here. Clinically detected when the glomerular filtration rate (GFR) falls below 60ml / min for at least three months, but it is not until it drops below 30ml / min that marked symptomatology occurs.

"Once the CRI has been detected, the diet becomes an unmatched strategy to help prevent or slow the deterioration of the kidneys, which is why what we eat and drink becomes important."

The recommendations of the diet of the person with CRF will vary depending on the stage and the characteristics of the disease itself. Still, they must take into account, necessarily, the following parameters:

Control of protein intake: A restriction of dietary proteins should be made because the substances derived from their metabolism (urea, creatine, phosphates) accelerate the evolution of the disease.

Sodium intake control: In renal failure, the kidneys are not able to remove excess sodium to maintain the body's balance. Also, sodium intervenes in our blood pressure and favours fluid retention, as well as causing a more excellent sensation of thirst, which can compromise fluid intake.

Control of potassium intake: Potassium is an essential mineral to maintain healthy nerve and muscle function. In renal insufficiency, the kidney is not able to eliminate the potassium that we ingest, being able to produce, if it accumulates in excess, muscular weakness, cramps, and even compromise our heart rate.

Phosphorus intake: Phosphorus is a mineral present in all foods, although in varying amounts. In renal failure, it accumulates in the blood and is responsible for vascular calcification and progressive deterioration of the bones.

Among these parameters, according to the state of the pathology, fluid intake should also be taken into consideration, so this intake should be adapted to the hydration and the diuresis state of the person, or, the nephrologist will determine the volume of fluid that can ingest.

One of the most common risks of this type of protein-restricted diet is malnutrition., with which we must ensure adequate caloric intake. To do this, taking into account the contribution of carbohydrates (the main component of food such as rice or fruit) that corresponds, will prove to be a good option — in this case, taking them in their refined version (for example, in flour, pasta, etc.), since the integral versions have high amounts of minerals, especially phosphorus. With the same purpose, lipids (usually called 'fats', are the main component of foods such as oil, butter, sauces such as mayonnaise, etc.), they will also provide us with calories, helping to enrich our diet. Still, it will be necessary to choose those rich in unsaturated fats (such as olive oil).

To facilitate that the intake of minerals with involvement in the pathology corresponds to the indicated restriction, it will be essential to know the content of these in foods, as well as their recommended consumption frequencies. Also, to reduce this mineral content of the foods to be consumed, it will be important to follow some recommendations on the cooking techniques used to prepare them. These culinary tips and recommendations will facilitate the elimination of a part of this mineral content so that the intake will be even lower.

For an adequate establishment of this type of food planning, the reading of nutritional labels will be very important, since they are usually a complete source of information that will allow us to choose the most suitable foods. Likewise, we must attend to the concept of ration, since it will be necessary to adjust the ratios of some food groups, with particular attention to proteins, and thus, not compromise health.

CHAPTER FOUR: Kidneys and Low-Carb Diet

Low carb is and will remain a much-discussed diet approach. While some see the best and healthiest weight loss strategy in a low-carbohydrate diet, others believe that low-carb is the direct route to heart attacks and vascular diseases. The truth will probably be somewhere in the middle, as is so often the case. However, a new study seems grist to the mill for low-carb critics. Because if you trust the results, a low-carbohydrate diet leads to kidney problems. The devil is in the details, however.

The downside of low carb diets

A mixture of scientific knowledge and clever marketing strategies set in motion a hysteria that sometimes takes on grotesque traits. With the carbohydrates, exactly that macronutrient is pilloried, which counts among its follower's huge amounts of vitamins and many minerals.

That renouncing carbohydrate leads to a comparatively rapid breakdown of body fat has meanwhile been proven several times and is considered a consensus among medical professionals, sports scientists, and nutrition experts alike. That said, that shouldn't hide the potential dangers of low-carb diets.

Why carbohydrates are so vilified

The foundation of the anti-carbohydrate movement is based on the knowledge that carbohydrates lead to the increased release of insulin. Insulin acts as an anabolic hormone the property of incorporating nutrients into our body tissue. Of course, this also includes the task of increasing our fat deposits whenever possible.

And that was exactly the fate of the carbohydrates because the supporters of Atkins and Co. carry the message into the world that the renouncement of carbohydrates hinders fat storage. Some advocates of the low-carb idea can even be carried away to say that this can completely prevent fat build-up.

The fact is, however, that carbohydrates only end up as belly fat or hip gold if you consume too much. However, this also applies to the other two macronutrients, namely proteins and fats.

Excessive meat consumption

Another disadvantage arises from the increased consumption of meat products and fats, which occurs automatically when the intake of carbohydrates is extremely restricted. It is not uncommon for dieters to confuse the low-carb approach with a free ticket for excessive meat consumption.

Due to the lack of carbohydrates, so the misconception, no fat can be stored anyway. Although there is some truth in this assumption, an excess of fat and protein calories, as intended by Mother Nature, is also built into our emergency stores.

Cholesterol levels rise

Besides, some low-carb people are not exactly health-conscious when preparing meat dishes. What good is shedding extra pounds if I get my cholesterol levels? Shedding buy levels that is beyond good and bad.

It is also a diabolical pact concerning purines, which promote the development of gout. It is best to go on a low-carbohydrate diet if you base it on lean meat, poultry, and fish.

CHAPTER FIVE: The Flawless 14-Day Renal Diet Meal Plan

Day 1

Morning: herbal tea to taste, wholemeal bread with low-fat quark, seasoned with freshly ground caraway seeds, paprika, turmeric

Lunch: pasta carrot pan with spring onions and pine nuts. To do this, cook the whole wheat ribbon pasta until soft, sauté the carrots and onions in a little safflower oil during the cooking time, then roast the pine nuts and add them. Mix everything on a large platter, season with fresh herbs such as parsley, and pour a few dabs of ricotta over the top.

Evening: oven vegetables. To do this, wash sweet potatoes, bell peppers, onions, garlic, potatoes, aubergines (choose according to your taste), cut into strips, and place on a tray greased with olive oil, bake at 200 degrees, season with fresh herbs such as rosemary. If that's too dry for you: Season skimmed yogurt with garlic and fresh dill and use as a dip.

In between / snack:

Fruit

Whole grain pastries, such as sesame pretzel, without the salt crumble

Green vegetable smoothie

Day 2

Morning: muesli made from oat flakes, some flaxseed, berries and low-fat yogurt, and herbal tea

Lunch: pasta salad with sun-dried tomatoes and oranges. Cook pasta such as farfalle or penne al dente, chop the dried tomatoes, and fillet an orange. Serve the tomato strips and orange fillets with a little olive oil, chop the fresh parsley or chervil and season the dressing with it, add fine fruit vinegar to taste, mix with the pasta.

Evening: tomatoes and cucumbers with mozzarella, flavoured with high-quality olive oil and fresh basil, served with whole-grain bread

In between / snack:

Fruit

Whole grain pastries, such as sesame pretzel, without salt crumble

Orange-red smoothie

Day 3

In the morning: Whole grain bread with cream cheese made from goat or sheep milk, seasoned with fresh herbs to taste, such as chives

Lunch: poultry steak with paprika vegetables (red, yellow, and green peppers, onions, some sour cream) and rice

In the evening: apple crumble. To do this, peel tart apples, cut into slices, and place in a lightly buttered baking dish. Drizzle with the juice of one lemon. From 100 grams of whole wheat flour, a handful of oat flakes, 80 grams of brown sugar and just as much butter, a pinch of cinnamon, knead a crumbly mixture and sprinkle it around the apples, bake in the oven at 200 degrees.

In between / snack:

Fruit

Whole grain pastries, such as sesame pretzel, without salt crumble

Green vegetable smoothie

Day 4

Morning: muesli and seasonal berries or apples, buckwheat flakes, oat milk

Noon: Italian bread salad. To do this, cut the ciabatta into slices, divide into bite-sized cubes, rub with a cut clove of garlic and moisten a little olive oil, briefly toast on a baking sheet in the oven, chop the tomatoes, cucumber, and onions for the salad and place in a large bowl. Prepare the vinaigrette from olive oil, balsamic vinegar, and many fresh herbs to taste, mix with the vegetables. Let the bread cool down briefly, fold into the salad and enjoy.

In the evening: vegetable soup (minestrone). Prepare vegetable broth from vegetables to taste - beans, zucchini, carrots, fennel, celery - first sauté the vegetables in olive oil, then fill up with a little water. Season with bay leaf, basil, and a pinch of salt (no more). Just before cooking, stir in a handful of soup noodles.

In between / snack:

Fruit

Whole grain pastries, such as sesame pretzel, without salt crumble

Red, rough and seasonal berries and banana smoothies, water

Freshly squeezed lemon juice, diluted with tap water

Day 5

In the morning: scrambled eggs from two eggs, pour over a diced tomato, season with fresh herbs, with wholemeal bread

Lunch: risotto with radicchio. To do this, sauté risotto rice in olive oil, add a finely diced onion and clove of garlic, fry briefly, pour a little vegetable stock, and cook over low heat. In another pan, sauté the sliced radicchio in olive oil, add a little salt, add a dash of oat cream and add this vegetable mixture to the risotto, fold in slightly. Season with fresh rosemary.

Evening: Baked vegetable stew. To do this, put the finely chopped vegetables of your choice in an ovenproof casserole dish with a lid, such as beans, pumpkin, tomatoes, courgettes, peppers, onions, kohlrabi. Add a cup of water, season with a little salt but a lot of herbs, if you like, also some chili, cover, and cook at 180 degrees for about 30 minutes. Then pour the ricotta flakes over the casserole and enjoy with the whole wheat baguette.

In between / snack:

Fruit

Whole grain pastries, such as sesame pretzel, without salt crumble

Green smoothie

Day 6

In the morning: Muesli made from millet, seasonal fruit, and rice milk

Noon: Salmon Pasta with lemon and zucchini. Sauté the salmon and zucchini in a little olive oil, add a little sour cream, season with lemon juice and a little salt. Boil the pasta and mix both, grind the pepper over it.

In the evening: sauté fried aubergines, aubergine slices, and onion slices in a little olive oil, flavour with lemon, add cherry tomatoes and capers to taste. Rice or whole-grain baguettes go well with it.

In between / snack:

Fruit

Whole grain pastries, such as sesame pretzel, without salt crumble

Green vegetable smoothie, for example, Lettuce, apple, and water with Romaine

Freshly squeezed lemon juice, diluted with tap water

Day 7

In the morning: whole grain bread with herbal cream cheese

Lunch: Tomatoes gnocchi. Make gnocchi from 500 grams of flour, boil potatoes, press a sieve or mash and knead with 125 grams of flour and egg, season with a pinch of salt and nutmeg. Shape the potato dough into rolls, cut tiny slices, press a fork on each piece, put in boiling water. When gnocchi float, they are done. Simply drizzle with liquid butter and flavour with fresh sage or serve with a simple tomato sauce (fresh tomatoes, onion, garlic, salt pinch, honey teaspoon). Gnocchi are excellent for freezing, so simply double and store in the freezer.

In the evening: asparagus with green vinaigrette, peeled green or white asparagus, boil, drain, prepare vinaigrette with olive oil, balsamic vinegar, and fresh herbs as desired. With wholemeal baguette.

In between / snack:

Fruit

Whole grain pastries, such as sesame pretzel, without salt crumble

Red smoothie, With (cooked) beetroot, apple, water

Freshly squeezed lemon juice, diluted with tap water

Day 8

Morning: herbal tea to taste, wholemeal bread with low-fat quark, seasoned with freshly ground caraway seeds, paprika, turmeric

Lunch: pasta carrot pan with spring onions and pine nuts. To do this, cook the whole wheat ribbon pasta until soft, sauté the carrots and onions in a little safflower oil during the cooking time, then roast the pine nuts and add them. Mix everything on a large platter, season with fresh herbs such as parsley, and pour a few dabs of ricotta over the top.

Evening: oven vegetables. To do this, wash sweet potatoes, bell peppers, onions, garlic, potatoes, aubergines (choose according to your taste), cut into strips, and place on a tray greased with olive oil, bake at 200 degrees, season with fresh herbs such as rosemary. If that's too dry for you: Season skimmed yogurt with garlic and fresh dill and use as a dip.

In between / snack:

Fruit

Whole grain pastries, such as sesame pretzel, without the salt crumble

Green vegetable smoothie, for example with kohlrabi and cucumber, water

Juice of one freshly squeezed lemon, diluted with tap water

Day 9

Morning: muesli made from oat flakes, some flaxseed, berries and low-fat yogurt, herbal tea

Lunch: pasta salad with sun-dried tomatoes and oranges. Cook pasta such as farfalle or penne al dente, chop the dried tomatoes, and fillet an orange. Serve the tomato strips and orange fillets with a little olive oil, chop the fresh parsley or chervil and season the dressing with it, add fine fruit vinegar to taste, mix with the pasta.

Evening: tomatoes and cucumbers with mozzarella, flavoured with high-quality olive oil and fresh basil, served with whole-grain bread

In between / snack:

Fruit

Whole grain pastries, such as sesame pretzel, without salt crumble

Orange-red smoothie, for example, Berries, oranges and carrots, water, water,

Freshly squeezed lemon juice, diluted with tap water

Day 10

In the morning: Whole grain bread with cream cheese made from goat or sheep milk, seasoned with fresh herbs to taste, such as chives

Lunch: poultry steak with paprika vegetables (red, yellow, and green peppers, onions, some sour cream) and rice

In the evening: apple crumble. To do this, peel tart apples, cut into slices, and place in a lightly buttered baking dish. Drizzle with the juice of one lemon. From 100 grams of whole wheat flour, a handful of oat flakes, 80 grams of brown sugar and just as much butter, a pinch of cinnamon, knead a crumbly mixture and sprinkle it over the apples, bake in the oven at 200 degrees.

In between / snack:

Fruit

Whole grain pastries, such as sesame pretzel, without salt crumble

Green vegetable smoothie, for example, Banana, cucumber, green lettuce, milk from rice

Freshly squeezed lemon juice, diluted with tap water

Day 11

In the morning: muesli with seasonal berries or apples, buckwheat flakes, oat milk

Noon: Italian bread salad. To do this, cut the ciabatta into slices, divide into bite-sized cubes, rub with a cut clove of garlic and moisten a little olive oil, briefly toast on a baking sheet in the oven. In the meantime, chop the tomatoes, cucumber, and onions for the salad and place in a large bowl. Prepare the vinaigrette from olive oil, balsamic vinegar, and many fresh herbs to taste, mix with the vegetables. Let the bread cool down briefly, fold into the salad and enjoy.

In the evening: vegetable soup (minestrone). Prepare vegetable broth from vegetables to taste - beans, zucchini, carrots, fennel, celery - first sauté the vegetables in olive oil, then fill up with a little water. Season with bay leaf, basil, and a pinch of salt (no more). Just before cooking, stir in a handful of soup noodles.

In between / snack:

Fruit

Whole grain pastries, such as sesame pretzel, without salt crumble

Smoothie red, About seasonal berries and bananas, water, etc.

Freshly squeezed lemon juice, diluted with tap water

Day 12

In the morning: whole grain bread with herbal cream cheese

Lunch: Tomatoes gnocchi. Make gnocchi from 500 grams of flour, boil potatoes, press a sieve or mash and knead with 125 grams of flour and egg, season with a pinch of salt and nutmeg. Shape the potato dough into rolls, cut tiny slices, press a fork on each piece, put in boiling water. When gnocchi float, they are done. Simply drizzle with liquid butter and flavour with fresh sage or serve with a simple tomato sauce (fresh tomatoes, onion, garlic, salt pinch, honey teaspoon). Gnocchi are excellent for freezing, so simply double and store in the freezer.

In the evening: asparagus with green vinaigrette, peeled green or white asparagus, boil, drain, prepare vinaigrette with olive oil, balsamic vinegar, and fresh herbs as desired. With wholemeal baguette.

In between / snack:

Fruit

Whole grain pastries, such as sesame pretzel, without salt crumble

Red smoothie, for example with (cooked) beetroot, apple, water

Freshly squeezed lemon juice, diluted with tap water

Day 13

In the morning: scrambled eggs from two eggs, pour over a diced tomato, season with fresh herbs, with wholemeal bread

Lunch: risotto with radicchio. To do this, sauté risotto rice in olive oil, add a finely diced onion and clove of garlic, fry briefly, pour a little vegetable stock, and cook over low heat. In another pan, sauté the sliced radicchio in olive oil, add a little salt, add a dash of oat cream and add this vegetable mixture to the risotto, fold in slightly. Season with fresh rosemary.

Evening: Baked vegetable stew. To do this, put the finely chopped vegetables of your choice in an ovenproof casserole dish with a lid, such as beans, pumpkin, tomatoes, courgettes, peppers, onions, kohlrabi. Add a cup of water, season with a little salt but a lot of herbs, if you like, also some chili, cover, and cook at 180 degrees for about 30 minutes. Then pour the ricotta flakes over the casserole and enjoy with the whole wheat baguette.

In between / snack:

Fruit

Whole grain pastries, such as sesame pretzel, without salt crumble

Green smoothie, With lettuce, pineapple, cucumber, and water, for example,

Freshly squeezed lemon juice, diluted with tap water

Day 14

In the morning: Muesli made from millet, seasonal fruit, and rice milk

Noon: Salmon Pasta with lemon and zucchini. Sauté the salmon and zucchini in a little olive oil, add a little sour cream, season with fresh lemon juice and a little salt. Boil the pasta and mix both, grind the pepper over it.

In the evening: sauté fried aubergines, aubergine slices, and onion slices in a little olive oil, flavour with lemon, add cherry tomatoes and capers to taste. Rice or whole-grain baguettes go well with it.

In between / snack:

Fruit

Whole grain pastries, such as sesame pretzel, without salt crumble

Green vegetable smoothie, With romaine lettuce, apple, and water, for example,

Freshly squeezed lemon juice, diluted with tap water

CHAPTER SIX: Breakfast Recipes

1. Papaya and cranberry jam

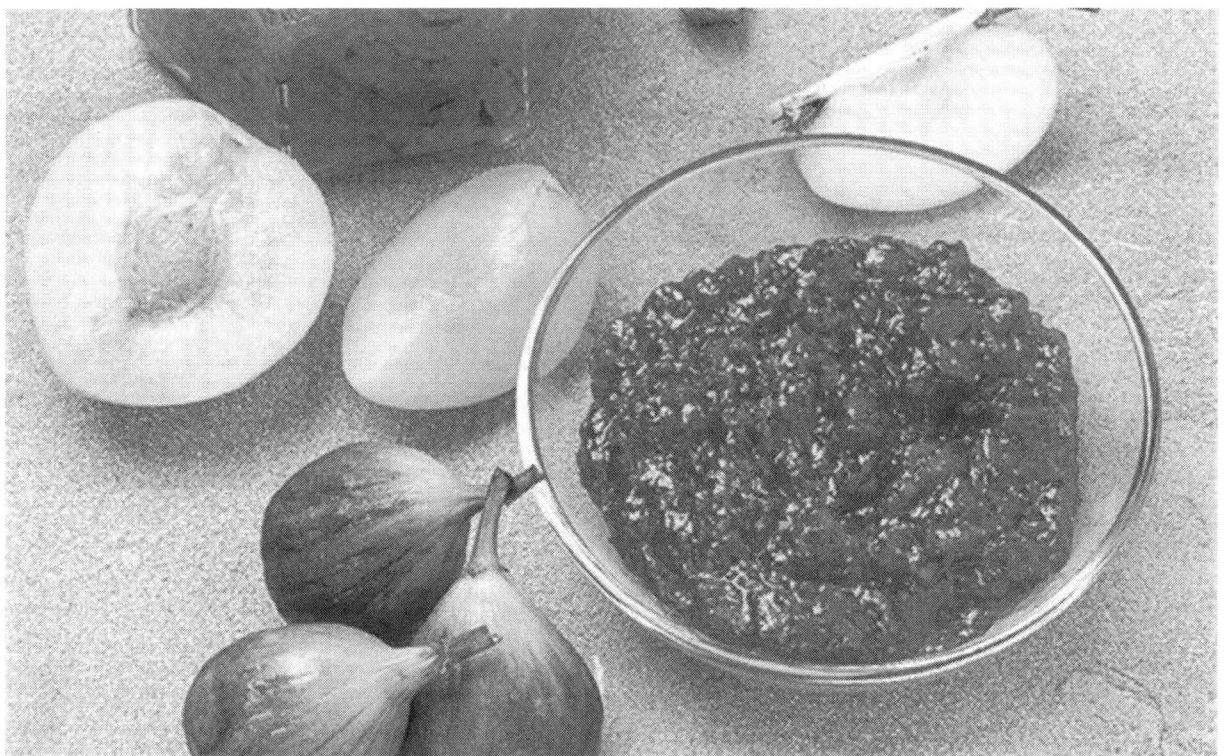

Total time 15mins, Preparation time 5mins, Serving 6

Ingredients:

- The pulp of a ripe papaya 700 grams
- Lemon juice 4 tbsp
- Cranberries / Cranberries 100 grams
- Preserving sugar 1: 1 1000 grams

Preparation:

1. With hot water, wash the papayas, rub them dry and peel them. Then cut it in half with a teaspoon and scrape the seeds out. With the lemon juice, purée the pulp. The cranberries are washed and sorted, put in a large saucepan, and lightly mashed with a fork. Add the papaya fruit puree and 1:1 of the gelling sugar and mix well.
2. While stirring, bring to the boil over high heat until all the food bubbles vigorously. Now the time for cooking begins! Let it simmer for 4 minutes, constantly stirring.
3. Remove the pot from the stove. Fill the hot mass quickly with jars rinsed with hot water to the brim and close immediately with the screw cap.

Nutritional information:

Information per 100g

kJ (kcal) 1440 (344), protein 0.1 g, carbohydrates 84.0 g, fat 0.1 g

2. Lemon curd

Preparation time: 5 minutes, Total time: 1 hour, 15 minutes (including cooling)

Ingredients:

- Freshly squeezed lemon juice 150 ml
- Freshly squeezed orange juice 100 ml
- Butter 100 gr.
- Sifted corn starch 30 gr.
- White wine dry 150 ml
- Sugar 150 gr.
- Grated lemon peel 1 pc.

Preparation:

1. Melt the butter and heat the corn-starch while stirring until it is light yellow. Add lemon and orange juice and the white wine. Please make sure that there are no lumps.
2. Now add the sugar and lemon zest and let it cook for another 2 minutes. Fill everything into glasses immediately.
3. The lemon curd unfortunately only lasts about 3 days in the refrigerator.

Nutritional information:

Information per 100g

kJ (kcal) 1000 (239), protein 0.3 g, carbohydrates 25.6 g, fat 12.9 g

3. Poor knight with apple compote

Total time 10mins, preparation time 15mins, serving 4

Ingredients:

- 4 large (or 8 small) slices of white bread
- 80 ml of cream
- 120ml water
- 1 egg
- 1 teaspoon vanilla pudding powder (for cooking)
- 2 tbsp sugar

- Breadcrumbs
- 40g butter
- Sugar and cinnamon to taste
- 400g apple compote

Preparation:

1. Mix the cream and water and stir together with the pudding powder, sugar, and egg until smooth. Halve or quarter the white bread slices and turn in the egg mixture.
2. Then turn in breadcrumbs and bake in hot butter over mild heat until golden brown on both sides.
3. Sprinkle with cinnamon sugar to taste and serve with the apple compote.

Nutritional values per serving:

Energy: 416kcal, Protein: 7g, Potassium: 192mg, Phosphate: 103mg

4. Pancakes with raspberries and ricotta

Total time 45mins, serving 2

Ingredients:

- 100g flour
- 1 egg
- 200 ml of mineral water
- 50ml cream
- 1 tsp baking soda
- 1 pinch of salt
- 2 tbsp rapeseed oil
- 80g raspberries
- 2 tbsp liquid honey
- 200g ricotta

Preparation:

1. Mix the flour with the egg, mineral water, cream, salt, and baking powder.
2. Let the dough rest for 10 minutes and fry 2 pancakes in hot rapeseed oil.
3. Fill with ricotta and raspberries and pour the honey over them.

Nutritional values per serving:

Energy: 575kcal, Protein: 21g, Fat:34g, Carbohydrates: 46g, Dietary fibre: 5g, Potassium: 294mg, Calcium: 265mg

5. Muesli made from rice flakes

Total time 10mins serving 2

Ingredients:

- 50 ml of cream
- 150 ml of water
- 2 tbsp sugar
- 35 g rice flakes
- 50 g blueberries from the glass, drained
- fresh mint

Preparation:

1. Bring the cream and water to the boil in a saucepan, then add the rice flakes and sugar, bring to the boil again briefly and remove from the stove. Let it soak for 10 minutes.
2. Divide between 2 bowls, add blueberries, and serve with the mint.

Nutritional values per serving:

Energy: 200kcal, Protein: 2g, Fat: 8g, Carbohydrates: 30g, Dietary fibre: 2g, Potassium: 68mg, Sodium: 10mg, Calcium: 32mg

6. Muesli mix, low in potassium

Ingredients:

- 200g millet flakes
- 150g corn flakes
- 150g rice crisps or puffed rice
- 50g desiccated coconut
- 50g sugar

Preparation:

1. Brown the coconut flakes with the sugar in a pan. Let cool and mix in the other ingredients. Store in a sealable jar.
2. Serve with a cream/water mixture and fruit compote (without juice) or quark.

Nutritional values per serving:

Energy: 231 kcal, Protein: 4g, Fat: 4g, Carbohydrates: 44g, Dietary fibre: 3g, Potassium: 67 mg, Calcium: 8 mg

7. Bamboo bread (low carb)

Serving 2

Ingredients:

- 150 g onions
- 1 tbsp olive oil
- 250 g low-fat quark
- 2 eggs
- 80 g of oat bran
- 25 g bamboo fibbers
- 30 g de-oiled gold flaxseed flour
- 1 teaspoon of tartar baking powder
- 1 teaspoon salt

Preparation:

1. Preheat the oven to 175 degrees (convection).
2. Peel the onions and cut into cubes. Heat the oil in a pan and gently fry the onion cubes for 5 to 6 minutes.
3. Then mix the onions well with all the other ingredients in a mixing bowl. Butter a rectangular baking pan or line it with baking paper. Pour in the batter and bake for 30-35 minutes. Let cool well before turning over.

Nutritional values per slice:

63 kcal, 3 g fat, 4 g carbohydrates, 5 g protein, 4 g fibber, 0.4 BE

8. Open bread with avocado

Serving 2

Ingredients (for 1 person):

- ½ avocado
- to taste: lemon juice
- 1 slice (40 g, e.g. spelled and rye) whole grain bread
- 200 g vegetables
- salt
- pepper

Preparation:

1. Peel the avocado and remove the stone. Drizzle the pulp with a little lemon juice, if you like, and either put it in fine slices on the wholemeal bread or mash with a fork and spread on the bread. Season with a little salt and pepper (fresh from the mill).
2. Wash the vegetables (for example some tomatoes, cucumber, paprika, and carrots), cut into small pieces, and serve as a raw vegetable side dish with bread.

Nutritional values:

304 kcal, 10 g protein, 15 g fat, 32 g carbohydrates, 14 g fibber

9. Bircher muesli with papaya

Prep time 5mins, total time 5mins, serving 2

Ingredients:

- 80 g crispy oat flakes
- 1 tbsp raisins
- ¼ l (1.5% fat) milk
- alternatively: ¼ l water
- 1 small (approx. 300 g) papaya
- 1 apple
- 150 g (1.5% fat) natural yogurt
- 2 teaspoons of lemon juice
- 1 tbsp pecan nuts
- 1 tbsp dried apple chips

Preparation:

1. Mix the oat flakes and raisins in a bowl with the milk (in the case of kidney stones, with water) the day before and leave to soak in the refrigerator for about 12 hours, preferably overnight.
2. The next day, cut the papaya in half, remove the core, peel and cut the pulp into 1-2 cm cubes. Wash the apple and grate finely around the core on a vegetable grater. Stir grated apple and half of the papaya cubes with the yogurt into the oatmeal mix. Finally, add the lemon juice to taste.
3. Spread the muesli mix on bowls. Roughly chop the pecans (omit if there are kidney stones) and sprinkle with the rest of the papaya. Serve garnished with the apple chips.

Nutritional values per serving:

420 kcal, 15 g protein, 11 g fat, 59 g carbohydrates, 9 g fibber, 280 mg calcium, 26 mg purine

10. Cauliflower and broccoli curry

Serving 2

Ingredients:

- 100 g chicken breast fillet
- 100 g cauliflower
- 100 g broccoli
- 1 tbsp rapeseed oil
- 1 tbsp curry powder
- 100 ml vegetable broth
- 100 ml coconut milk

Preparation:

1. Wash the meat, pat it dry and dice it. The vegetables should be washed and cleaned and cut into small florets. Instead of being fresh, frozen vegetables can also be used.
2. In a bigger pan, heat the oil, fry the meat cubes for approximately 2 minutes and add the vegetables. Briefly fry and stir in the powder with the curry. Add the coconut milk and vegetable stock, and simmer for 8-10 minutes. Put a bit of salt to taste if necessary.

In the case of rosacea, choose a mild curry powder and dose it carefully. If necessary, season only with turmeric and coriander.

Nutritional values:

463 kcal, 34 g fat, 10 g carbohydrates, 30 g protein, 8 g fibbers

11. Broccoli and lentil salad with mackerel

Preparation time 10mins, total time 20mins serving 2

Ingredients:

- 300 g broccoli
- 1 small onion
- 4 tbsp orange juice
- 2 tbsp white wine vinegar
- 2 tbsp olive oil
- salt

from the mill: pepper

- 1 teaspoon (from the jar) grated horseradish

- 1 can (240 g drained weight) lentils
- 125 g of cocktail tomatoes
- 4 stalks of basil
- 2 smoked (approx. 150 g, skin-on) mackerel fillets

Preparation:

1. Wash and cut the broccoli into florets, peel the stalks and cut into small cubes. Peel the onion and cut into fine cubes.
2. In a small saucepan, bring the onion cubes to the boil with orange juice, vinegar, and olive oil. Add the broccoli and cook covered over medium heat for about 3 minutes. Remove from heat and season with salt, pepper, and horseradish.
3. Rinse the lentils in a sieve and let them drain well. Wash and halve the tomatoes. Gently mix the lentils and tomatoes into the broccoli.
4. Wash the basil, pat dry, and pluck the leaves. Peel the mackerel fillets and cut into bite-sized pieces. Cover the salad with the mackerel pieces, sprinkle with basil, and season with pepper.

Nutritional values per serving:

380 kcal, 17 g protein, 27 g fat, 13 g carbohydrates, 6 g fibbers, 1 BE

12. Broccoli rice gratin (Italian Style)

Total: 1 hr 15 mins, Prep: 30 mins, serving 2

Ingredients:

- 125 g (10-minute) brown rice
- salt
- 300 g broccoli florets
- 200 g of strained (canned) tomatoes
- salt

from the mill: pepper

- 1 teaspoon dried Italian herb
- 1 teaspoon (noble sweet variety) paprika powder
- 100 g cocktail tomatoes
- 125 g (8.5% fat) small mozzarella balls
- 2 tbsp pine nuts
- some basil leaves

Preparation:

1. As per the instructions on the packet, cook the rice with plenty of salted water. Meanwhile, clean the broccoli florets and wash them, and cut them into smaller pieces. Add the broccoli to the rice about 5 minutes before cooking time ends, bring it all to a boil again, and simultaneously cook the broccoli.
2. Preheat the oven to 220 ° C. Grease a baking dish (20 x 30 cm approx.) with oil. Drain in a colander with the rice and broccoli and drain. Use salt, pepper, Italian herbs, and paprika powder to season the tomatoes. Mix and dissolve in the baking dish with the broccoli rice mix.
3. Wash and slice the cherry tomatoes in half. Halve the balls of mozzarella as well. Combine the tomatoes and mozzarella, sprinkle with the pine nuts, and spread on the broccoli-rice mix. On the middle rack, bake the gratin in the oven for about 10 minutes. To serve, sprinkle with the basil leaves.

Nutritional values per serving:

320 kcal, 18 g protein, 15 g fat, 26 g carbohydrates, 6 g fibbers, 145 mg calcium, 45 mg purine

13. Colorful bean salad

Total: 10, Prep: 10mins, serving 4

Ingredients:

- 200 g green beans
- 1 onion
- 1 bell pepper
- 1 small can (drained weight 250 g) white beans
- 1 small can (drained weight 250 g) kidney beans
- 2 tbsp wine vinegar
- 2 tbsp sour cream
- 1/2 teaspoon mustard
- 1/2 teaspoon tomato ketchup
- 1/2 teaspoon horseradish
- salt
- pepper
- 1 tbsp oil
- chopped thyme

Preparation:

1. Clean and wash the green beans and cook in salted boiling water for 6-8 minutes until they are firm to the bite. Pour into a sieve, rinse in cold water and drain well. Transfer to a large bowl.
2. Peel the onion and cut into thin rings. Halve and core the peppers lengthways, wash and cut into cubes. Drain the kidney beans and white beans each into a sieve, rinse with cold water and drain well. Then add the onion, bell pepper, kidney beans, and white beans to the green beans.
3. For the dressing mix together vinegar, sour cream, mustard, tomato ketchup, horseradish, oil, and thyme, season with salt and pepper. Mix with the salad ingredients and let the bean salad steep for about 5 minutes before serving.

Nutritional values (per serving):

210 kcal, 7 g protein, 11 g fat, 15 g carbohydrates, 6 g fibber

14. Fennel and Orange Salad

Prep: 10 mins, Total: 10 mins, serving 4

Ingredients:

- 1 small ripe banana
- 200 g cream
- 2 tbsp walnut oil
- 1-2 teaspoons (from the jar) horseradish
- alternatively: freshly grated horseradish
- to taste: tarragon
- salt
- from the mill: black pepper
- 2 small fennel bulbs
- 2 small apples
- 2 oranges
- some freshly squeezed lemon juice
- 10 walnut halves

Preparation:

1. Mash the banana with a fork and mix with the cream, oil, horseradish, and possibly a little tarragon to make a salad dressing. Add salt and pepper to taste.
2. wash the fennel and cut into very fine strips. Wash the apples, remove the core, and dice very finely (do not peel). Drizzle the fennel and apples with a little freshly squeezed lemon juice and add to the sauce.

3. Peel the oranges, cut out the individual fillets and add them to the sauce with the roughly chopped walnuts. Mix everything and serve chilled.

Nutritional values (per serving):

345 kcal, 5 g protein, 25 g fat, 25 g carbohydrates, 6 g fibbers

15. Fruity egg salad

Total time 25mins, preparation 10mins, serving 4

Ingredients:

- 8 eggs
- 4 tbsp (4.8% fat) mayonnaise
- 6 tbsp (1.5% fat) yogurt
- 2 tbsp white wine vinegar
- 2 tsp curry
- if you like: cayenne pepper
- salt and pepper
- 2 tart apples
- 2 tbsp fresh parsley
- 1 red onion
- 4 pickles
- 2 tbsp sunflower seeds

Preparation:

1. Boil the eggs hard for 8 minutes. Then rinse in cold water and let cool down. In the meantime, for the dressing, mix the mayonnaise in a bowl with the yogurt, vinegar, curry, cayenne pepper, salt, and pepper if you like.
2. Wash the apples carefully or (if not organic) peel, core, and cut into medium-sized cubes. Wash and finely chop the parsley. Peel the onion and cut into thin rings. Cut the pickled cucumbers into fine cubes. Peel the cooled eggs and cut them into cubes.
3. Mix the apple, parsley, onion, cucumber, and eggs in a large bowl and stir in the mayonnaise dressing. Serve the egg salad sprinkled with sunflower seeds. A slice of wholemeal bread tastes good with it.

Nutritional values (per serving):

330 kcal, 19 g protein, 16 g fat, 24 g carbohydrates, 3 g fibber

16. Baked mushrooms with pollock cream cheese

Preparation time 15mins, total time 30mins, serving 4

Ingredients:

- 30 g Alaska pollock
- 1 splash Lemon juice
- 10 large mushrooms
- 4 tsp black (without stone) olives
- 300 g cream cheese
- 2 tbsp olive oil
- salt
- pepper
- at will: Italian herbs
- some chili powders

Preparation:

1. Preheat the top and bottom heat of the oven to 150-200 degrees (180 degrees of circulating air) or heat the garden grill.
2. Rinse the fish fillet, pat dry, slice the escalope into thin pieces and mix with the lemon juice. Remove the stems, clean the mushrooms and chop them into small cubes. Cut the olives into thin slices.
3. With the finely chopped mushroom stalks, the olive rings, the saithe schnitzel, and the oil, mix the cream cheese. Season with salt, chili powder, and pepper. Place the mushrooms in a baking dish or grill tray and pour the cream cheese mixture into the mushrooms. For about 20 minutes, cook.

Nutritional values per serving:

663 kcal, 60 g fat, 5 g carbohydrates, 25 g protein, 3 g fibber, 0.4 BE

17. Quinoa oat muesli

Preparation time 5mins, total time 30mins, serving 1

Ingredients:

- 1 pear
- 3 tbsp quinoa flakes
- 1 tbsp oatmeal
- 3 tbsp natural yogurt

- 1 tbsp chopped cashew nuts
- 1 tbsp sunflower seeds
- alternatively: 1 tbsp chopped dried fruit

Preparation:

1. Wash the pear, cut into quarters, remove the core, and roughly dice.
2. Put the quinoa and oat flakes together with the yogurt in a bowl, sprinkle with pear pieces and the seeds, or the chopped dried fruit.

If you prefer a smooth porridge, you can also put all the ingredients in a powerful mixer. Depending on your tolerance, you may omit cashew and sunflower seeds.

Nutritional values:

279 kcal, 9 g protein, 6 g fat, 44 g carbohydrates, 8 g fibers

18. Quark breakfast with mango

Total time 5mins, preparation time 5mins, serving 2

Ingredients:

- 1 mango
- 500 g low-fat quark
- 6 tbsp Oat drink
- 2 tbsp linseed
- 2 tsp Flea seeds
- 2 tbsp Sunflower seeds
- 2 tbsp linseed oil

Preparation:

Peel the mango off the stone and remove the pulp. Place in a mixing bowl together with all other ingredients and purée until smooth with the mixer.

Nutritional values per serving:

431 kcal, 18 g fat, 25 g carbohydrates, 40 g protein, 8 g fibber, 2.1 BE

19. Blueberry Pancakes

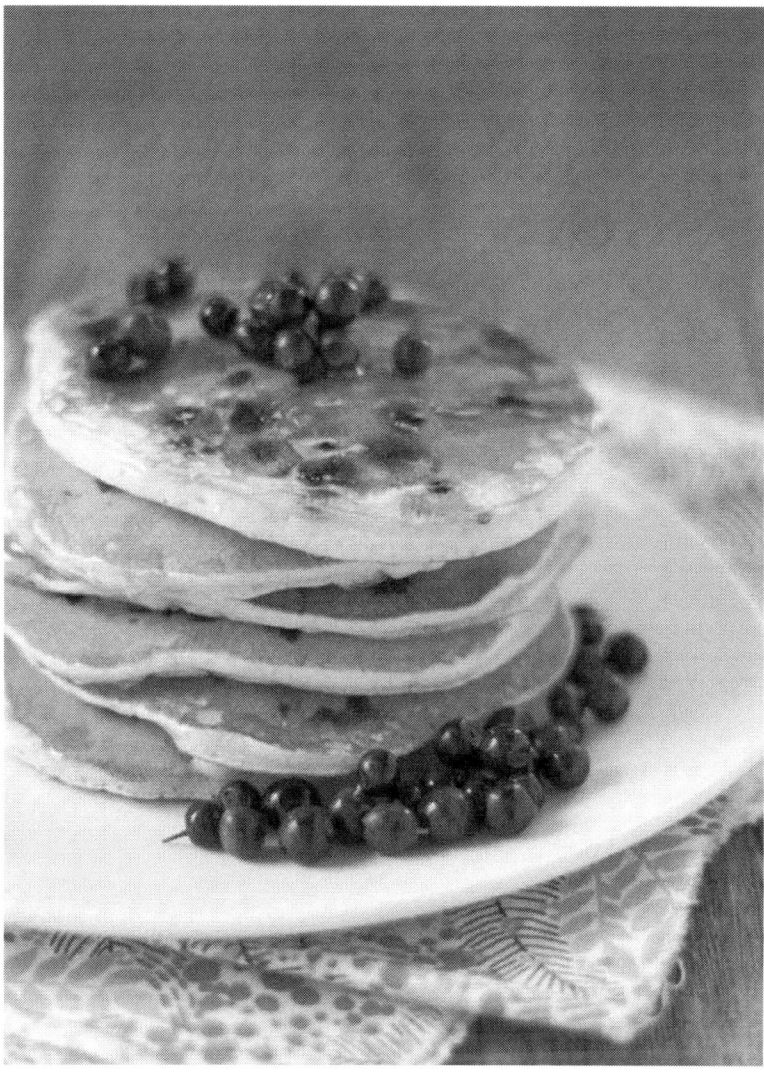

Total time 15mins, preparation time 5mins, serving 2

Ingredients:

- 2-3 cups of flour
- 2 teaspoons baking powder
- 3/4 cup flaked oatmeal
- 1/4 cup sugar
- 1 3/4 cup milk (more or less depending on taste)
- 2 eggs
- 20 grams of melted butter
- 1 tablespoon vanilla extract
- a pinch of salt
- Blueberries at ease

Preparation:

1. Mix the flour, baking powder, oatmeal, pinch of salt, and sugar.
2. Add milk, egg yolks, melted butter, vanilla extract.
3. Raise the egg whites to the point and add them to the mixture in an envelope.
4. Cook in a bowl and add the blueberries to each pancake.
5. Serve with maple honey.

Nutritional information:

146.3 calories; Protein 5.1 g 10%; Carbohydrates 24.7 g 8%; Fat 2.9 g 5%; Cholesterol 36.8 mg 12%; Sodium 397.4 mg 16%.

20. Banana Breakfast Pancakes

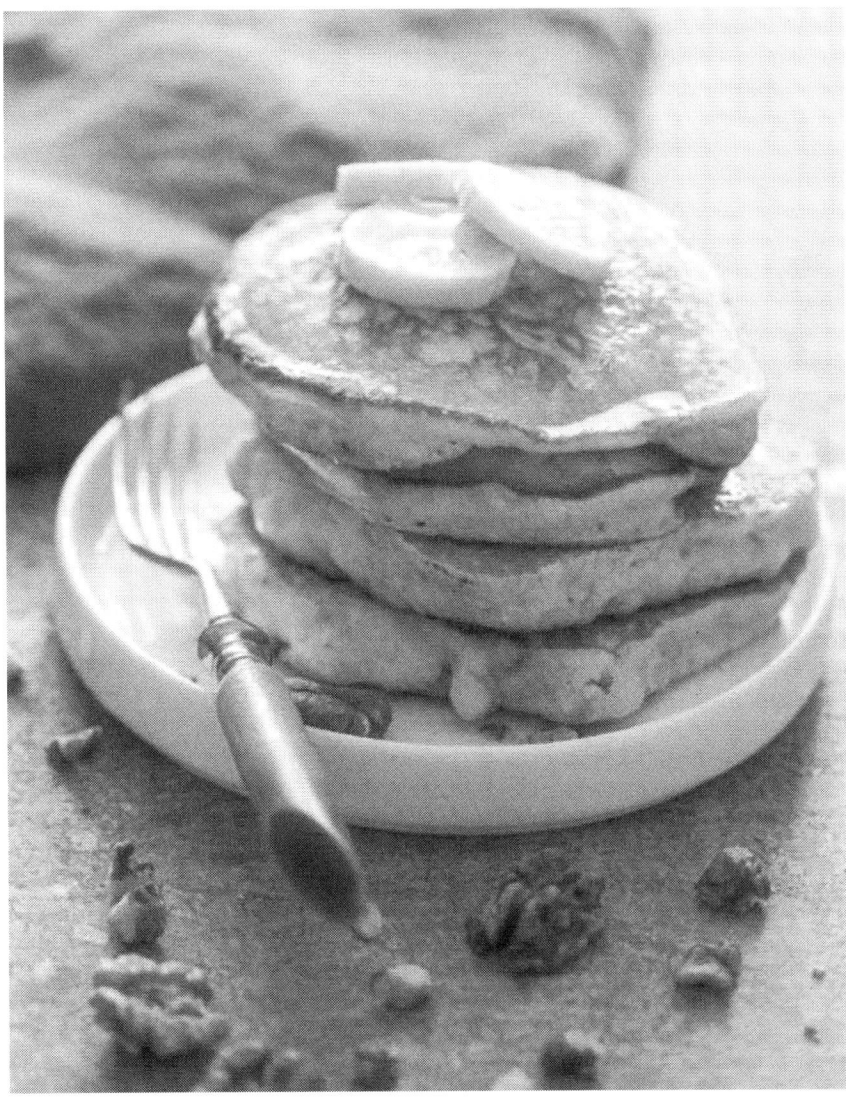

Total time 10mins, preparation time 5mins.

Ingredients:

- ½ cup (63g.) Of wheat flour.
- ½ cup (80g.) Of flaked oatmeal.
- 2 small bananas (160g.) Mashed.
- 2 eggs (100g.).
- 1 cup (240g.) Ideal, 0% Fat, Evaporated Milk.
- 2 tablespoons (30g.) Brown sugar.
- 1 tablespoon (6g.) Of cinnamon.
- 1 teaspoon (5g.) Of butter.

Preparation:

1. In a big basin, combine all ingredients, except butter.
2. In a pan over medium heat, place the butter and wait for it to melt.
3. Pour ¼ cup of the mixture over the pan and cook until it begins to bubble.
4. Turn the pancake and cook for 1 minute or until it browns on the other side.
5. Serve and enjoy.

Nutritional values per serving:

Calories: 484 Kcal, Fats: 7 g, Saturates: 3 g, Carbs: 87 g, Sugars: 19 g, Fibbers: 5 g, Protein: 15 g, Salt: 1.21 g

21. Tuna Spinach Sandwich

Total time 10mins, preparation time 10mins, serving 2

Ingredients:

- The quantity of ingredients is to your liking and preference.
- Integral bread
- Fresh and well-washed spinach
- Tuna in well-drained water
- A ripe but firm avocado
- Salt and pepper

Preparation:

1. The spinach already washed and dried the short in thin strips, the finest you can.
2. What I do to achieve these strips is, I arrange several spinach leaves on top of each other, I make a small roll, and with a very sharp knife, I am cutting and thus they are excellent.

3. Avocado cut it into tiny cubes.
4. The bread is browned in a Teflon pan, on one side only.
5. Mix spinach with tuna and avocado.
6. Season the mixture with salt and pepper.
7. You put the stuffing in the bread and go.
8. Enjoy this delight.

Nutritional Information:

Calories: 157 Total Fat: 7g Saturated Fat: 4g Cholesterol: 44 Mg Sodium: 422 Mg fibbers: 1g Sugar: 3g Protein: 21g

22. Cranberry Quinoa Salad

Total time 30mins, preparation 10mins

Ingredients:

- 1 1/2 cups of water
- 1 cup raw quinoa, rinsed
- 1/4 cup chopped red pepper
- 1/4 cup yellow pepper, chopped
- 1 small red/purple onion, finely chopped
- 1 1/2 teaspoons curry powder
- 1/4 cup chopped fresh cilantro
- 1 lemon, juiced
- 1/4 cup toasted sliced almonds
- 1/2 cup chopped carrots
- 1/2 cup dried cranberries
- Salt and ground black pepper to taste.

Instructions:

1. Pour the water into a casserole dish and cover it with a lid. Boil over high heat, then pour the quinoa, recover and continue over low heat for 15 to 20 minutes until the water has been absorbed. Transfer to a mixing bowl and chill until cold in the refrigerator.
2. Red pepper, yellow pepper, onion, curry powder, cilantro, lemon juice, sliced almonds, carrots, and blueberries should be added when cold. Season with salt and pepper to taste. Before serving, relax.

Nutritional Information:

Calories: 218 Total Fat:8g Saturated Fat:1g Cholesterol:0Mg Sodium:60Mg Carbohydrates: 33g fibbers: 4g Sugar: 12g Protein: 5g

CHAPTER SEVEN: Poultry and Meat Recipes

23. Summer pot pie

Serving: 4

Ingredients:

- 1 onion, finely chopped
- 2 carrots, peeled and diced
- 1 cup (250 mL) green beans cut into 1/2-inch (1 cm) chunks or 1 cup green peas.
- ¼ cup (60 mL) canola oil
- 2 boneless, skinless chicken breast halves, cubed
- 2 garlic cloves, finely chopped
- ¼ cup (60 mL) unbleached all-purpose flour
- 2 cups (500 mL) low sodium chicken broth
- 1 cup (250 mL) small cauliflower florets
- ¼ cup (60 mL) chopped flat-leaf parsley
- 4 oz (115 g) frozen phyllo dough, thawed and cut into ½ slices cm (¼ inch) thick (see note)
- 2 Tbsp. (30 mL) canola oil
- Pepper to taste

Preparation:

1. Put the grill in the oven centre. Preheat oven to 180 ° C (350 ° F).
2. Soften the onion, celery, carrots, and beans in the oil over medium heat for about 8 minutes.
3. Add chicken, cook until lightly browned. Pepper, guy. Reduce medium-heat temperatures. Add garlic and cook for 1 minute.
4. Sprinkle well with flour. Add the chicken stock and cook, stirring with a whisk. Simmer for 2-3 minutes.
5. Add parsley and chopped flowers and mix well. Adjust seasoning. Place in a 20-cm (8-inch) baking dish. Book it.
6. Spread the strips of phyllo dough and drizzle on a baking sheet. Mix gently. Spread the pell-mell over the mixture without pressing.

Nutritional values:

Energy: 358 g, Protein: 21 g, Carbohydrates: 22 g, fibbers: 2.3 g, Total Fat: 21 g, Sodium: 188 mg, Phosphorus: 187 mg, Potassium: 432 mg

24. Grilled turkey with lime

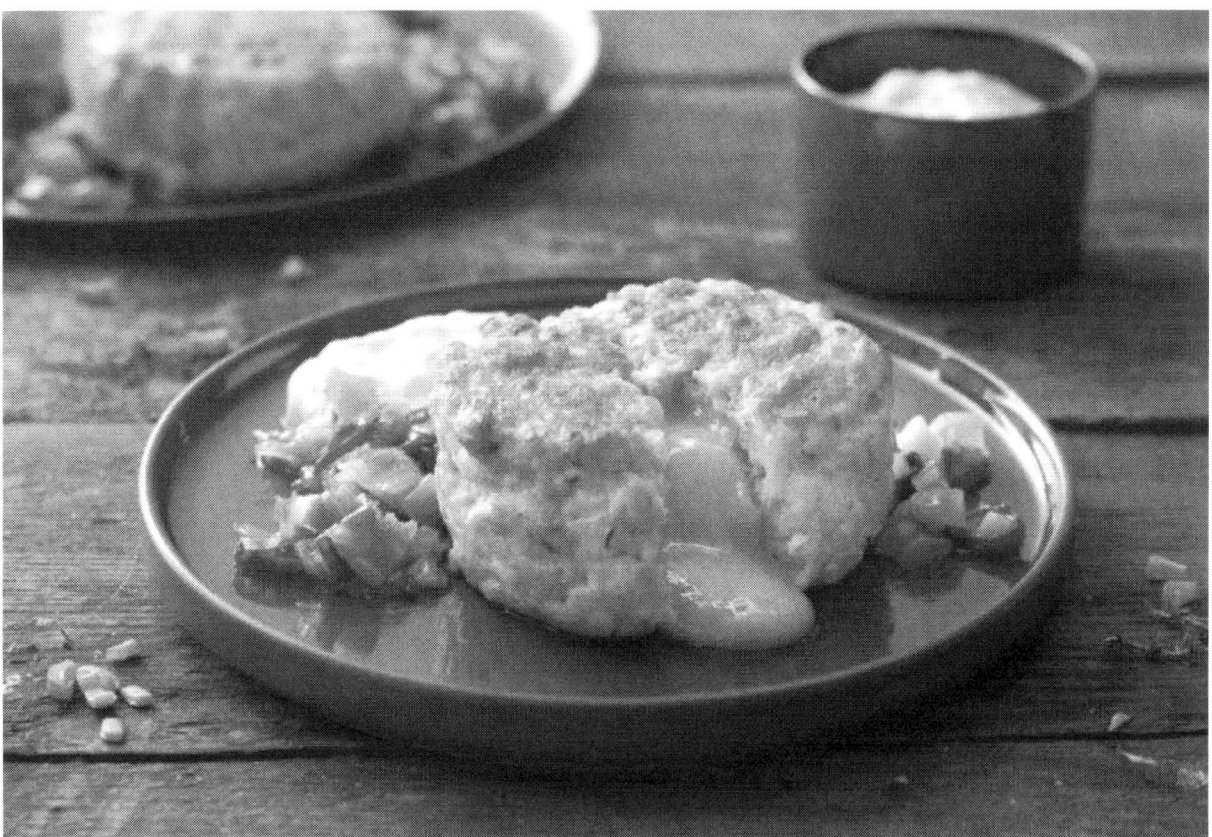

Serving 4

Ingredients:

- ½ cup (125 mL) Lime juice
- ¼ cup (60 mL) Vegetable oil
- 2 tbsp. (30 mL) Liquid Honey
- 1 Tbsp. (5 mL) Dried Thyme Leaves
- 1 tsp. (5 mL)
- 2/3-pound dried rosemary (300g) Turkey breast, skinless, boneless

Preparation:

1. Prepare the marinade by mixing the first five ingredients.
2. Reserve 2 tbsp. (30mL) marinade for brushing.
3. Cut the breast into two thick slices to make cutlets.
4. Add the cutlets to the marinade. Cover and refrigerate 1 - 2 hours.
5. Preheat the broiler on high power (500 ° F) or preheat the barbecue.
6. Remove the breast from the marinade.
7. In the oven or on the barbecue, grill the cutlets for 4 minutes per side or until cooked through.

8. Use the reserved marinade to brush the cutlets during cooking.
9. Discard the rest of the marinade.

Nutritional values:

Energy: 245 g, Proteins: 17.1 g, Carbohydrates: 11.5 g, fibbers: 0.4 g, Total Fat: 15 g, Sodium: 35 mg, Phosphorus: 131 mg, Potassium: 200 mg

25. Curry turkey casserole

Serving 4

Ingredients:

- ¼ cup and 2 tbsp. canola oil or olive oil
- 1 small yellow onion, diced
- 2 garlic cloves, minced
- ¼ cup all-purpose flour
- 1 cup of 2% milk
- 2 cups no salt added chicken broth
- 2 tbsp. curry powder
- pepper
- 3 cups of broccoli heads
- 1 cup chopped red peppers
- 4 cups cooked turkey cut into ¾ inch pieces
- 3 cups of bread cut into medium cubes

Preparation:

1. Preheat oven at 400 ° F. Heat 1/4 cup of canola oil or olive oil over medium heat. Add garlic and onion. Cook until tender, but about 7 minutes before turning golden. With a whisk, add flour and stir with a whisk for a minute. Add milk and chicken broth slowly, whisking constantly until the mixture is smooth. Cook, stirring frequently until the sauce cooks. Add curry powder and season with pepper. Add broccoli heads and cook until broccoli begins to tender, about 5 minutes. Adding the turkey. Pour into an 8-inch square baking dish.
2. Pour 2 tbsp into a bowl. Canola or olive oil on bread cubes and coat evenly. Transfer the bread cubes to the turkey mixture and cook in the oven until bubbly and golden brown, about 15 minutes.

Nutritional values:

Energy: 380 g, Protein: 26 g, Carbohydrates: 23 g, fibbers: 2 g, Total Fat: 20 g, Sodium: 113 mg, Phosphorus: 227 mg, Potassium: 472 mg

26. Grilled Chicken Salad

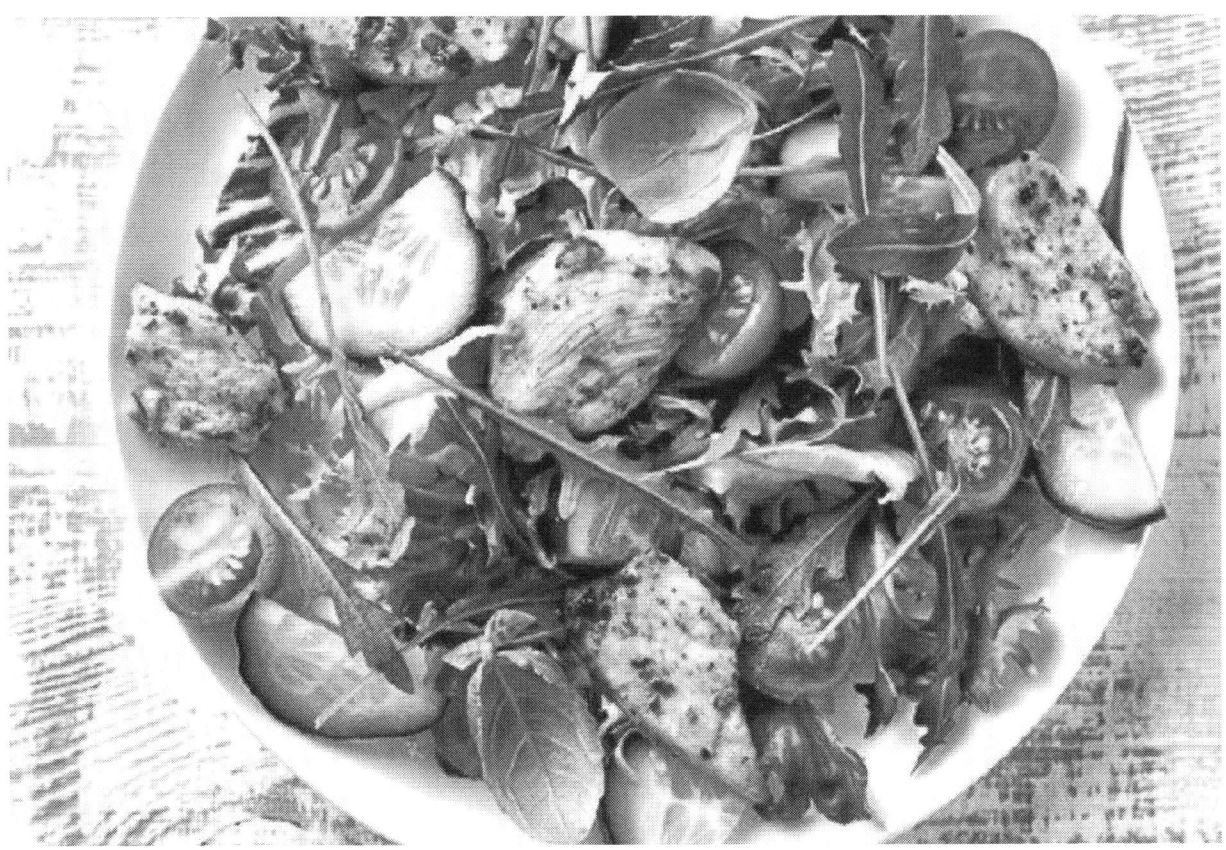

Ingredients:

- 4 boneless skinless chicken breast (s)
- 1 Tbsp. (5 mL) soy sauce
- 2 tbsp. (30 mL) extra virgin olive oil
- 2 tbsp. (30 mL) cilantro, fresh, fresh
- 1 Tbsp. (15 mL) ginger, minced
- 2 garlic cloves
- 1/2 tsp. (2.5 mL) hot pepper flakes
- 2 yellow bell pepper (s), large
- 3 tbsp. (45 mL) rice vinegar
- 5 1/2 cups (1.375 L) mesclun salad

Preparation:

1. Mince the coriander or fresh coriander. Combine soy sauce, half oil, cilantro, ginger, and garlic in a large bowl. Cover the chicken breasts well. Cover and marinate in the refrigerator for 30 minutes or up to a day.

2. Meanwhile, quarter the peppers. Preheat grill to medium. Grill the peppers for about 15 minutes or until black. Remove from heat, place on a plate. Place the chicken breasts on the greased grill and cook 10-15 minutes per side over medium heat or until a thermometer inserted into the breasts reads 165 ° F (74 ° C).
3. Grilled peppers and chicken in 1/2-inch strips. Combine chicken, peppers, and salad in a salad bowl. Add remaining oil and vinegar.

Nutritional values:

Energy: 380 g, Protein: 26 g, Carbohydrates: 23 g, fibbers: 2 g, Total Fat: 20 g, Sodium: 113 mg, Phosphorus: 227 mg, Potassium: 472 mg

27. Makhani Chicken

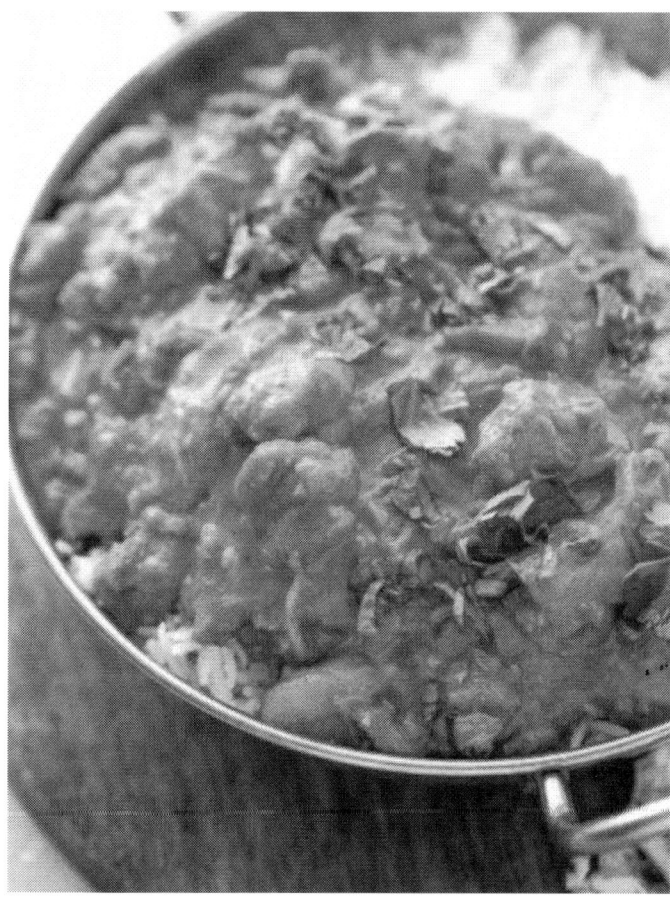

Serving 4

Ingredients:

Chicken

- 1 lb (454 g) boneless skinless chicken thighs, cubed
- 1 tbsp. to s. oil

- 1 onion
- 2 slices of ginger
- 2 cloves of garlic
- 2 cups unsalted tomato puree
- 1/2 cup yogurt
- 1 tsp. at t. ground cumin
- 2 tbsp. at t. garam masala
- 1/4 tsp. at t. cayenne pepper (optional)
- 1/2 cup chopped cilantro

Flavoured Basmati Rice

- 1 cup Basmati rice
- 1 tsp. at t. olive oil
- 1 bay leaf
- 1/2 tsp. at t. turmeric
- 1 1/2 cups water
- Cardamom
- Cinnamon stick

Preparation:

Chicken

1. Crush the onion, ginger, and garlic in a blender
2. Heat 1 tbsp. to s. of oil. Sauté the mixture with the cumin, cayenne pepper (optional), and 1 tsp. at t. garam masala.
3. Add the tomatoes and cook for 2 minutes, stirring frequently.
4. Stir in the yogurt and simmer for 10 minutes at low temperature, stirring frequently. Remove from the heat and set aside.
5. Heat 1 tbsp. to s. of oil, add the chicken and brown it. Pour in a few spoons of the sauce, and simmer until the sauce reduces and the meat is no longer pink. Add the chicken to the sauce. Add the coriander.
6. Cook for 5-10 minutes over low heat. Stir from time to time.

Flavoured Basmati rice

1. Heat the oil in a saucepan.
2. Add the rice and spices and lightly toast the mixture.
3. Add water. Boil the water.
4. Cover and simmer for about 15 minutes.

Nutritional values per serving:

Calories/Energy: 295 Kcal, Carbs: 13.7 g (19%), Lipids: 15.4 g (46%), Protein: 26.2 g (35%), Fibbers: 2.7 g, Salt: 0.69 g, Cholesterol: 76 mg, Potassium: 635 mg

28. Moroccan chicken

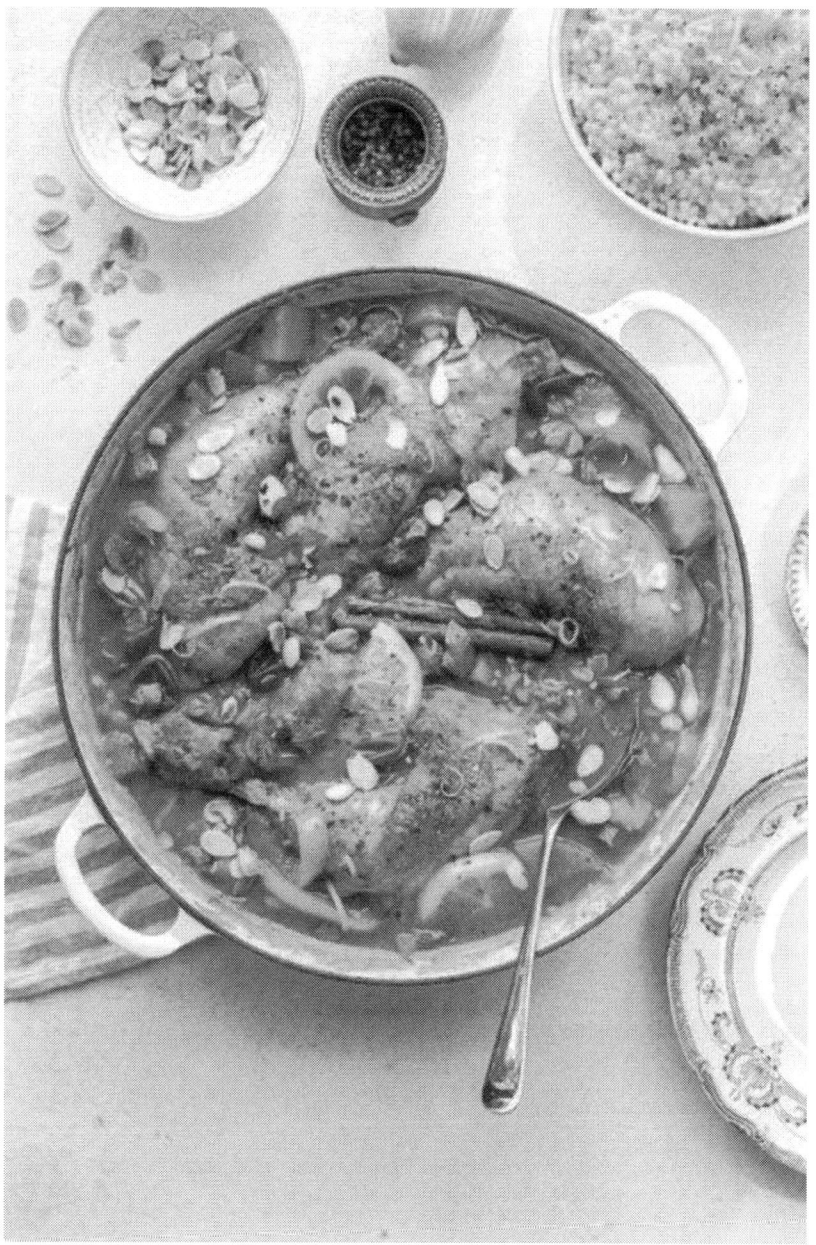

Serving 4

Ingredients:

- 1/3 cup of honey
- 1 teaspoon of sesame oil
- 2 tablespoons of lemon juice

- ½ teaspoon of lemon zest
- 3 cloves of garlic, crushed
- ½ teaspoon of ground cumin
- 1 teaspoon of paprika
- ¼ teaspoon onion powder
- ¼ teaspoon of cinnamon
- ¼ teaspoon of nutmeg
- ½ teaspoon of cayenne pepper
- ¼ teaspoon of black pepper
- 6 chicken breasts or thighs with the bone and skinless

Preparation:

1. Combine the first 12 ingredients and add the chicken to marinate.
2. Refrigerate between 1 and 24 hours, remembering to turn the pieces from time to time.
3. Line a baking sheet with foil. Arrange the chicken on the foil, bone side down. Pour the extra marinade over the chicken.
4. Bake at 400 ° F for 30 to 40 minutes or until the chicken is cooked through.

Nutritional values:

Energy: 196 g, Protein: 26 g, Carbohydrates: 16 g, Total Fat: 3 g, Sodium: 79 mg, Phosphorus: 218 mg, Potassium: 305 mg

29. Chicken stuffed with herbs and ricotta cheese

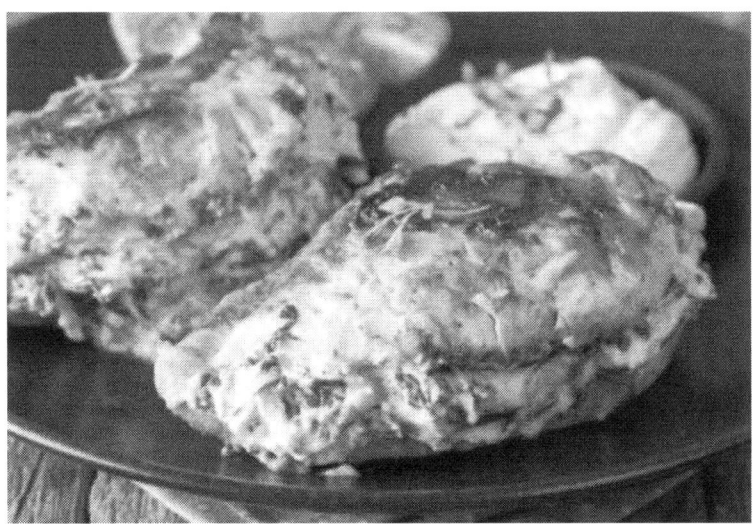

Ingredients:

- 1 garlic clove, sautéed
- 1 tbsp. to s. extra virgin olive oil

- cups ricotta cheese
- 1 egg
- ¼ cup chopped herbs
- ¼ tsp. at t. black pepper
- 2 large (6 ounces each) chicken breasts (boneless and skinless)

Preparation:

1. Brown the garlic in olive oil.
2. Combine the ricotta cheese, egg, garlic, and herbs.
3. Slit the thickest part of the chicken breast.
4. Insert the stuffing into the chicken breast.
5. Heat the olive oil in a pan.
6. Brown the chicken in the pan and transfer it to the dish to put it in the oven heated to 350 ° F.
7. Cook for 20 to 30 minutes.

Nutritional values:

Energy: 277 g, Protein: 32 g, Carbohydrates: 5 g, Total Fat: 13 g, Sodium: 181.5 mg, Phosphorus: 387 mg, Potassium: 353 mg

30. Chicken salad with cranberries and tarragon

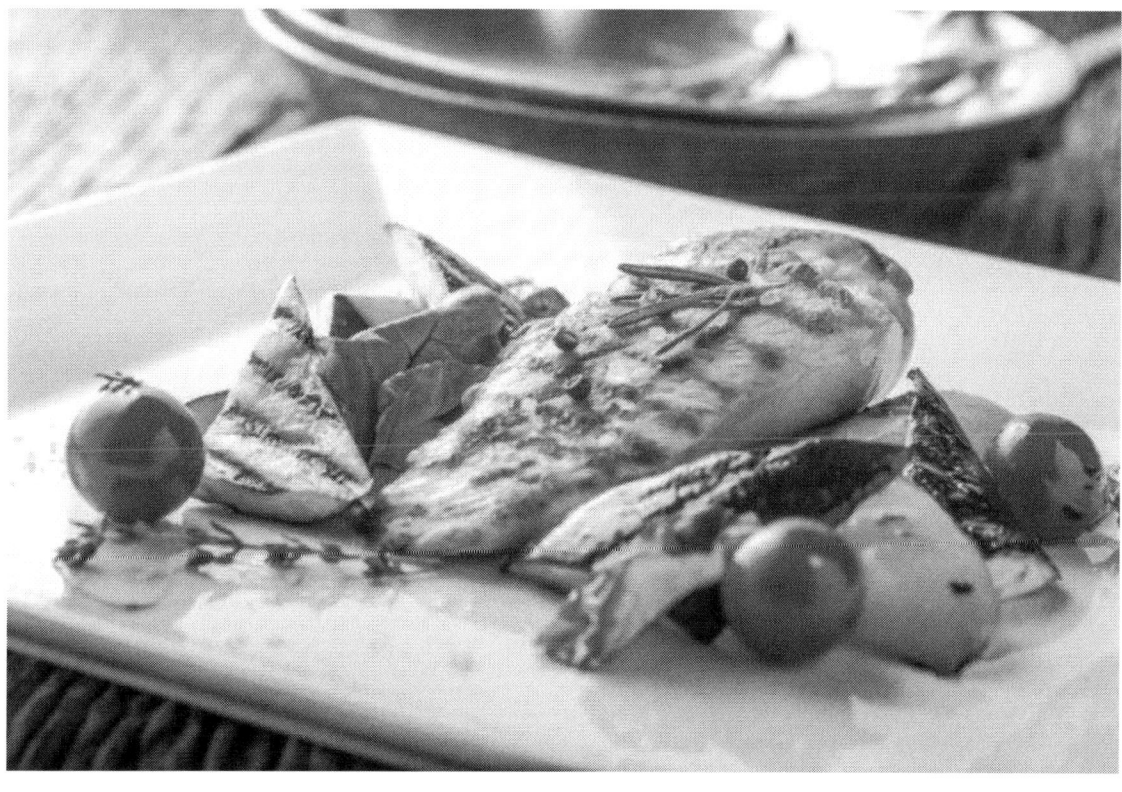

Serving 4

Ingredients:

- 2 cups minced cooked chicken
- ¼ cup finely chopped dried cranberries
- 1 Tbsp. minced French shallot
- 1 tbsp. lemon juice
- ¼ cup mayonnaise
- 1 tsp. teaspoon minced fresh tarragon
- 1 tsp. black pepper
- 8 slices white bread

Preparation:

1. In a basin, combine all the ingredients except the bread.
2. Make 4 sandwiches with the bread and salad, pressing gently on the slices.

Nutritional values:

Energy: 368 g, Protein: 26.5 g, Carbohydrates: 42 g, fibbers: 2 g, Total Fat: 9 g, Sodium: 443 mg, Phosphorus: 233 mg, Potassium: 258 mg

31. Roast beef meatloaf with protein-free bread

Serving: for one low-protein portion

Ingredients:

- 400 grams of lean beef, minced
- 2 slices of protein-free bread (about 35 g)
- 50 ml of protein-free milk
- 20 gr of grated Parmesan cheese (about 2 tablespoons)
- 1 whole egg
- 25 grams of flour
- A pinch of salt
- (FOR THE COOKING)
- 20 gr of butter
- 20 gr of oil
- 2 sprigs of rosemary
- A few sage leaves
- 1 glass of dry white wine

Preparation:

1. Remove the crust from the slices of bread, break them up in a bowl, sprinkle them with milk and squeeze them eliminating the excess milk.
2. Add the meat, working the mixture with your hands to mix the two ingredients well, add the grated Parmesan, egg, and salt, continuing to work the mixture until it is perfectly homogeneous.
3. Form the meatloaf and pass it in the flour. Put a pan on the fire, which you can then put in the oven, and heat oil and butter with the aromatic herbs. Add the meat and brown it until it is well coloured, add the wine letting it evaporate in half, and then pass in a hot oven at 180 ° -200 ° for about 1 hour. If it gets too dry, add a drop of wine and cover the pan with aluminium foil.
4. Let the meat cool before cutting it into thick slices.

It's possible to reduce, even if minimally, the protein intake by using protein-free bread and milk in the dough of this meatloaf.

Nutritional values:

Protein: 24 g, Calories: 298 kcal, Potassium: 7 *, High Phosphorus, Lipids: 18 g, Cholesterol: 133 mg

32. Pork loin with herbs

Serving 1 - 4

Ingredients:

- Pork loin about 500 gr
- Rosemary 4-5 sprigs
- Sage 5-6 leaves
- Coriander 1 tablespoon of seeds
- Jamaica pepper 1 tbsp
- Black pepper 1 tsp
- Coarse salt 1 tsp
- 2 cloves garlic
- 2 tablespoons extra virgin olive oil
- (FOR THE DRESSING)
- Pitted green olives about 20
- Marjoram a little fresh leaves
- 1 fresh chili
- 2 tablespoons extra virgin olive oil

Preparation:

1. Cut the loin into a couple of places to insert the garlic cloves (for those who cannot tolerate it, it is certainly possible to skip this step).
2. Chop both herbs and spices, including coarse salt, in a blender.
3. Place the meat in a baking dish and cover it with the mince making it adhere well so that cooking creates a crust. Drizzle with a drizzle of extra virgin olive oil and put in the oven at 230 ° for the first 15 minutes, then lowering to 200 ° for another 30 minutes.
4. When cooked, turn off the oven and leave the meat in it for a few more minutes with the oven open.
5. Remove from the oven and let it cool completely. If possible, prepare the roast the day before and store it in the refrigerator wrapped in aluminium foil.
6. To serve: slice the meat as thin as possible, just over a slice of ham, arrange it on a serving dish and sprinkle it with coarsely chopped olives, marjoram leaves, thinly sliced chili, and a drizzle of extra virgin olive oil.

Note on allspice: the round balls, widely used in Caribbean cuisine, are appreciated for their particular taste (intense and aromatic, not very spicy), which looks like a mixture of different spices. The flavour is reminiscent of cinnamon, black pepper, clove, and nutmeg combined. The composite aroma therefore justifies the appellation of 'all spices' that this berry receives in English (allspice) and in French (toute-épice).

Nutritional values:

Protein: 25 g, Calories: 280 kcal, Potassium 13 *, Very High Phosphorus, Lipids: 20 g, Cholesterol: 76 mg

33. Zucchini cream with chicken

Serving 1 - 4

Ingredients:

- 300 g of already cleaned zucchini
- 200 g of chicken breast
- 100 g of natural yogurt
- 2 bay leaves
- 1 shallot
- 7 basil leaves
- 20 g of extra virgin olive oil
- a pinch of salt
- a grind of pepper

Preparation:

1. Wash the courgettes and cut them into small pieces, removing any internal seeds. Put them in a saucepan full of cold water with 2 bay leaves and the shallot cut in 4. Boil for about 15-20 minutes.
2. Once cooked, drain the zucchini with the shallot, keeping a little of their cooking water in case it is needed to reduce the density, and blend with the basil and yogurt.
3. In the meantime, you have cut the chicken breast into bite-sized pieces and roasted it in a non-stick pan for about 10 minutes. When cooked, add salt and pepper.
4. Pour the zucchini cream into small bowls, add the chicken nuggets and garnish with a few basil leaves, a drizzle of oil, and a grind of pepper.

Remember that, for dishes like this, the double boiling of the vegetables helps to reduce the potassium values by about 1/3.

Nutritional values:

Protein: 12 g, Calories: 117 kcal, Potassium 7 *, Low Phosphorus, Lipids: 7 g, Cholesterol: 38 mg

34. Beef carpaccio

Serving: for one portion of about 100 g

Ingredients:

- 100 g of beef slices for carpaccio
- 1 tablespoon of lemon juice
- 1 tablespoon of extra virgin olive oil
- a modest pinch of salt
- a grind of pepper
- 20 g of rocket

Preparation:

1. Have the butcher cut the meat into very thin slices.
2. Arrange them on a flat plate, sprinkle them with lemon juice and finish the seasoning with salt, pepper, and oil.
3. Serve it with the rocket salad.

To remain within acceptable values, I've eliminated Parmesan, which in the classic recipe accompanies carpaccio, allowing tasting this dish for those who love raw meat.

Nutritional values:

Protein: 21 g, Calories: 221 kcal, Potassium 8 *, Medium Phosphorus, Lipids: 15 g, Cholesterol: 60 mg

35. Low-protein fusilli with meat sauce

Serving: 1 - 4

Ingredients:

- 300 gr of protein-free fusilli
- A pinch of salt
- (FOR THE MEAT SAUCE)
- 200 gr of minced beef pulp
- 50 gr of onion
- 50 gr of celery
- About 100 g of peeled and seeded ripe tomatoes
- 15 gr of butter
- 1 tablespoon of extra virgin olive oil
- 1 small pinch of salt
- 4-5 tablespoons of grated Parmesan cheese

Preparation:

1. Chop the onion and celery and fry them over moderate heat with the oil. Then add the minced meat and a modest pinch of salt and cook until it has cleared and dried up; then add the peeled tomatoes and two ladles of hot water. Cover and bring to the boil. Then adjust the heat to low and cook for about an hour, stirring often and adding water if necessary.
2. Separately, cook the fusilli, then season with the meat sauce and raw butter, adding the cheese lastly.
3. As a general rule, it is best to reduce the amount of cheese.

The use of protein-free paste must be prescribed by the nephrologist.

Nutritional values:

Protein: 15 g, Calories: 418 kcal, Potassium 6 *, Medium Phosphorus, Lipids: 11 g, Cholesterol: 48 mg

36. Ginger Chicken

Serving: 1 - 4

Ingredients:

- 200 g of low protein rice
- 400 g of chicken breast
- 1 dry chili
- Juice of one lemon

- 50 g of fresh ginger
- 100 g of skimmed yogurt
- 1 clove of garlic
- 20 g of raisins
- 1 tablespoon of coriander seeds

Preparation:

1. Rub the chicken breasts with the lemon juice emulsified with the chopped chili. Let it rest in the refrigerator for 30 minutes.
2. Blend the yogurt with the garlic, raisins, peeled and grated ginger, and dried coriander.
3. Place the chicken in a bowl and cover it with the marinade, letting it rest in the refrigerator for at least 12 hours.
4. Bake the chicken in the oven at 200 ° for about 30 minutes, making sure that it is always moistened by the marinade.
5. Serve it hot accompanied by the protein-free rice that you have boiled according to the package directions.

Tonic, digestive and anti-inflammatory, this is ginger. A spice with great healing properties that can characterize even the simplest dishes.

Nutritional values:

Protein: 21 g, Calories: 318 kcal, Potassium 9 *, Medium Phosphorus, Lipids: 5 g, Cholesterol: 77 mg

37. Beef stew with rice

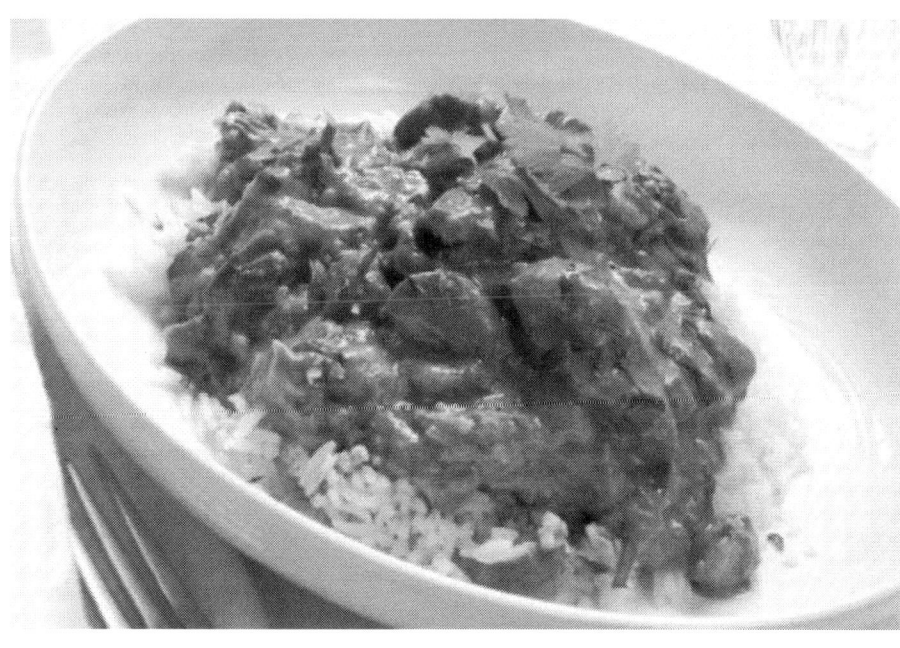

Serving: 4

Ingredients:

- Lean beef rump 400 g
- Extra virgin olive oil 40 g
- Onion 100 g
- Tomato 300 g
- Rosemary
- Sage
- Garlic
- Juniper berries
- Rice 200 g
- Water 400 cc
- Extra virgin olive oil 10 g
- Little onion

Preparation:

1. Cut the beef into small pieces and put it in a saucepan with the herbs and oil. Cook over low heat for about half an hour adding water and wine as required. Then add the ripe tomato and cook for at least another hour.
2. Meanwhile, prepare the pilaf rice. Finely chop the onion and sauté it on low heat in oil with a few tablespoons of water. Add the rice, toast, and then add the water.
3. Cover making sure that the lid does not allow steam to escape. Cook with the lid on for the time indicated on the rice package.

Single dish suitable for dialysis patients. If you have potassium problems you cannot add the tomato: the stew is good anyway! Sodium is that contained in food. Use them according to your diet.

Nutritional values:

Water: 276 g, Protein: 27 g, Phosphorous: 301 mg, Potassium: 605 mg, Lipids: 15 g, Carbs: 42 g, Sodium: 55 mg, Calories: 409 kcal

CHAPTER EIGHT: Lunch Recipes

38. Chick Curry (Thai Chicken)

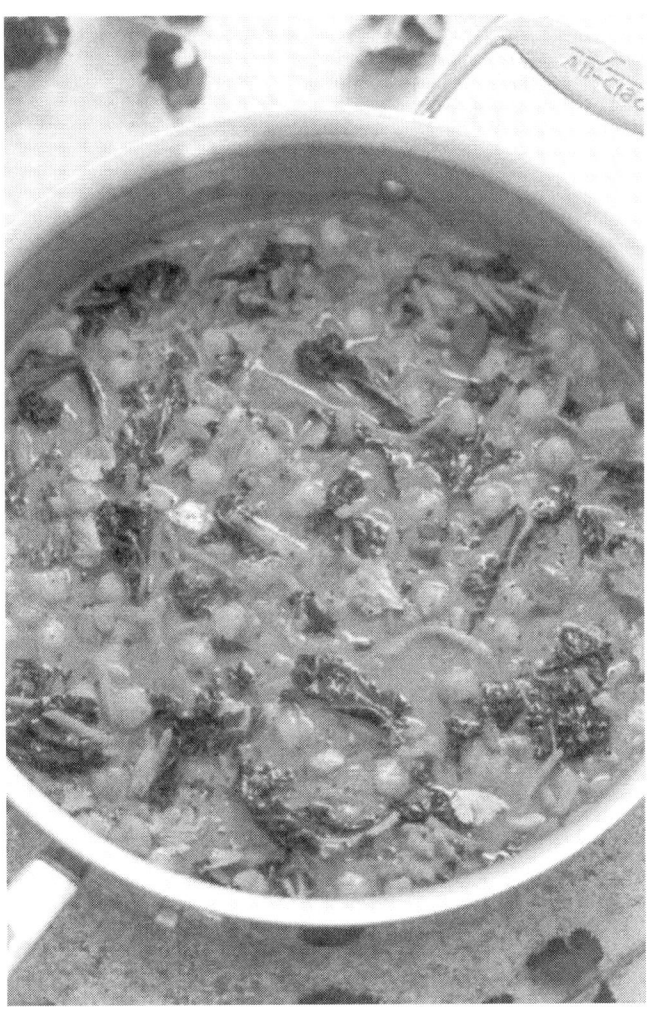

Preparation time 30mins, total time 30mins, serving 4-6

Ingredients:

- 2 skinless, boneless chicken breasts (not too small)
- 3 tablespoons olive oil
- 1 small onion, finely chopped
- 2 cloves garlic, minced
- 3 tablespoons curry powder
- 1 teaspoon ground cinnamon
- 1 teaspoon paprika
- 1 bay leaf
- 1/2 teaspoon freshly grated ginger root

- 1 tbsp tomato extract
- 1 bottle of coconut milk
- 1/2 lemon (juice)
- 1 red bell pepper
- 1 cup pineapple (optional)

Preparation:

1. In a basin season the chicken cubes with salt and lemon juice and set aside.
2. Put in a pan the olive oil, garlic, onion, and fry until golden brown.
3. Then put the chicken in the pan and fry until golden brown.
4. Add pineapple (optional), curry, cinnamon, paprika, bay leaf, tomato extract, ginger, and red pepper. Fry for a few more minutes (if necessary, add a cup of water).
5. Add coconut milk, cook for a few more minutes and serve.

Nutritional information:

295.2 calories; Protein 19.1 g 38%; Carbohydrates 19.2 g 6%; Fat 16.9 g 26%; Cholesterol 43.1 mg 14%; Sodium 352.9 mg 14%.

39. Fried breaded lasagna with marinara sauce

Total Time 4 hr 22 min, Prep Time 10 minutes, serving 4-6

Ingredients:

- 6 large slices of lasagna
- 1 cup of ricotta or cottage cheese
- 1 cup of mozzarella cheese
- 3 eggs
- ½ tablespoon of Italian seasoning
- 1 tablespoon of chopped parsley
- 1 clove of crushed garlic
- salt and pepper
- ¼ cup wheat flour
- c / n breadcrumbs
- c / n vegetable oil

Directions:

1. Cook in a large saucepan with water before the lasagna, according to the manufacturer's instructions.
2. Place the lasagna sheets on a previously greased baking sheet.

3. Combine ricotta cheese, mozzarella cheese, 1 egg, Italian seasoning, parsley, garlic and salt, and pepper to taste in a bowl. Incorporate all ingredients very well.
4. Distribute the previous mixture on each of the lasagna sheets and roll very well by pressing the filling.
5. To breach, pass each lasagna roll through bowls of flour, bowl with 2 beaten eggs, and to finish the dish with the breadcrumbs. Then enter the freezer for 30 minutes.
6. Heat oil in a deep pan. Introduce the lasagna rolls one by one and fry for 2 to 3 minutes. Place on the paper towel to remove the excess oil.
7. Cut lasagna rolls in half and serve on a marinara sauce base.

Marinara sauce:

1. In a medium saucepan heat 2 tablespoons of oil, add 1 finely chopped onion and 1 clove of crushed garlic, and brown for 5 minutes.
2. Stir with a wooden spoon to prevent burning. Add 2 cups of chopped tomato, 2 tablespoons of tomato paste, and 2 tablespoons of chopped fresh basil, ½ tablespoon of ground black pepper, 1 teaspoon of ground oregano, and ½ tablespoon of salt.
3. Cook until the sauce boils. Put it on low heat and continue cooking for 20 minutes or until the sauce acquires a thick consistency.

Nutritional values per serving:

Calories/Energy: 207 Kcal, Lipids: 7 g, Carbs: 25 g, Protein: 11 g, Water: 56 g

40. Baked Mushrooms with Pumpkin and Chipotle Polenta

Ingredients:

- 900 g mix of mushrooms, such as maitake, jasmine ear, and black shimeji - coarsely chopped - thinly sliced porcini crimini mushrooms - and coarsely chopped shiitakessem stalks
- 1/3 cup of extra virgin olive oil
- 1 garlic head, crushed cloves
- A small handful of sage, finely chopped or sliced
- Sea salt and freshly ground black pepper.
- 1 cup cooked pumpkin puree
- 3 cups chicken broth
- Nutmeg, freshly grated
- 1 chipotle adobo sauce, seedless and finely chopped, plus a small spoon of adobo sauce
- 1 cup quick-cooking polenta
- 2 tbsp butter
- 2 tbsp honey

- Roasted seeds for decoration
- Chives, minced, for decoration

Preparation:

1. Preheat the oven to 220 ºC.
2. Mix the mushrooms with extra virgin olive oil, garlic, brine, salt, and pepper and bake for 25 minutes.
3. Meanwhile, in a small pan, put it pumpkin puree over medium heat, along with some chicken broth to dilute.
4. Season with salt, pepper, and nutmeg.
5. In another pan, put the remaining stock and bring to a boil, then add the chipotle, adobo sauce, polenta and mix using a wire whisk. Continue beating the polenta until the sides are far from the pan walls, then add the butter, honey, and beat again.
6. Combine pumpkin and polenta and serve in individual shallow bowls.
7. Top with roasted mushrooms and Siva with roasted seeds and chives for garnish.

Nutritional values:

Calories/Energy: 324 Kcal, Lipids: 1 g (3%), Carbs: 64.9 g (84%), Protein: 9.8 g (13%)

41. Quinoa salad with chickpeas and feta

Cooking time: 15 min, Total Time: 35 minutes, serving 4

Ingredients:

- 1 onion
- 1 toe garlic
- 1 tbsp olive oil
- 150 ml vegetable broth
- 100 g Quinoa
- 60 g Feta
- 215 g (Drained weight, from the jar) chickpeas
- 1 small bunch of coriander
- 0.5 lemon
- Salt
- Pepper
- 0.5 tsp Ras el Hanout

Preparation:

1. Peel and finely chop the onion and garlic, sauté in a saucepan with oil. Deglaze with the vegetable stock, bring to the boil and cook the quinoa in it according to the instructions on the packet.
2. In the meantime, pour the chickpeas out of the glass into a sieve, rinse and drain. Wash the coriander, shake dry and chop. Squeeze the lemon. Prepare a dressing from lemon juice, salt, pepper, Ras el Hanout and coriander.
3. Put the finished quinoa in a bowl, pour the drained chickpeas and the dressing over it. Finally, crumble the feta and mix it with the quinoa salad. Let it steep for at least 15 minutes. The salad tastes lukewarm or cold.

Nutritional values (per serving):

469 kcal, 20 g protein, 20 g fat, 52 g carbohydrates, 9 g fibbers

42. White Bean Salad

Serving 2

Ingredients:

- ½ cucumber
- 1 bunch of rockets
- 1 can (200 g) giant white beans
- 1 red pepper
- 3 spring onions
- 3 tbsp white balsamic vinegar
- Salt
- Pepper
- 1 teaspoon honey
- 4 tbsp olive oil

Preparation:

1. Drain the beans in a colander. Wash the cucumbers, cut in half, core, and cut into slices. Wash the rocket and spin dry. Wash, core, and cut the peppers into small cubes. Wash and clean the spring onions and cut into rings.
2. Whisk the balsamic vinegar, salt, pepper, honey, and olive oil together.
3. Mix the lettuce, vegetables, and beans in a bowl and carefully fold in the dressing.

Nutritional values per serving:

282 kcal, 20 g fat, 18 g carbohydrates, 4 g protein, 4 g fibbers

43. Omelette and summer vegetables

Serving 1

Ingredients:

- Non-stick cooking spray
- 1/4 cup of frozen whole kernel corn, thawed
- 1/3 cup chopped zucchini
- 3 tablespoons chopped green onion
- 2 tablespoons water
- 1/4 tsp of black pepper
- 2 large egg whites
- 1 large whole egg
- 1-ounce low-fat sharp cheddar cheese

Preparation:

1. Heat a cup over medium-high heat. Coat with cooking spray.
2. Add corn, zucchini, and onions to the pot; sauté 4 minutes or until tender and firm.
3. Remove fire. Heat a 10-inch pan over medium-high heat. Combine in a bowl water, pepper, egg whites, and egg, mix well with a whisk.
4. Coat with cooking spray.
5. Pour the egg mixture into the bowl; cook until edges are set (about 2 minutes).
6. Gently lift the omelette edges with a spatula, tilting the pan to bring the uncooked egg mixture into contact with the pan.
7. Sprinkle the vegetable mixture with cheese using a spoon on one half of the omelette.
8. Using the spatula, peel the omelette and fold the omelette back (in half).
9. Cook two more minutes or until melted. Slide the omelette onto a plate.

Nutrient Analysis:

Energy: 187 g, Protein: 22 g, Carbohydrates: 11 g, fibbers: 1.6 g, Total fat: 6 g, Sodium: 270 mg, Phosphorus: 218 mg, Potassium: 352 mg

44. Elderberry asparagus with herbal cream cheese

Cooking time: 30 min, total time 1 h 50 min, serving 4-6

Ingredients:

- 1 kg white asparagus
- 3 tbsp butter

- 4 tbsp elderflower syrup
- salt
- 5 elderflower umbels
- 500 g waxy potatoes
- 10 g mint (0.5 bunch)
- 300 g cream cheese
- 150 g yogurt (3.5% fat)
- pepper
- 1 tsp lemon juice
- 10 g parsley (0.5 bunch)
- 10 g chives (0.5 bunch)

Preparation steps:

1. Peel the asparagus and the woody ends are cut off. With 1 tbsp of butter, grease a baking dish and place the sticks in it. Season with salt, sort the elderflower, and spread on the asparagus. Drizzle with the syrup. Cover the tin and cook the asparagus for 60–80 minutes in a preheated oven at 100 ° C (fan oven: 80 ° C; gas: level 1).
2. Peel and wash the potatoes and cook in salted boiling water for 25–30 minutes.
3. Wash the mint, shake it dry, and chop the leaves finely. Mix the yogurt with the cream cheese, mix in the mint, and season with salt, pepper, and lemon juice.
4. Wash and dry the parsley, shake and chop. In a pan, heat the remaining butter, drain the potatoes, allow them to evaporate, and toss the butter and parsley in the hot pan.
5. Wash the chives, shake them dry, then cut them into rolls. Take the asparagus out of the oven with the flower umbels, arrange 4 plates with the parsley potatoes and the mint cream cheese, and serve sprinkled with chives.

Nutritional values:

Calories 543 kcal (26%), Protein 18 g (18%), Fat 36 g (31%), Carbohydrates 37 g (25%)

45. Soup of green asparagus

Cooking time: 40mins, total time 60mins, serving 2

Ingredients:

- 250 g green asparagus
- 1 shallot
- 10 g butter (1 tbsp)
- 400 ml classic vegetable broth
- 30 g parmesan (1 piece)

- ½ lemon
- 4 tbsp soy cream
- salt
- pepper
- 100 ml milk (1.5% fat)
- 3 drops truffle oil

Preparation steps:

1. Wash and drain the asparagus and cut off any woody ends. Peel the asparagus in the lower third. Cut the sticks into pieces about 2 cm long. Peel and finely chop the shallot.
2. Heat the butter in a saucepan. Sauté the asparagus pieces and shallot in it over medium heat.
3. Pour in the vegetable stock and bring to the boil. Cook on low heat for about 15 minutes.
4. In the meantime, grate the parmesan cheese finely.
5. Add the parmesan to the asparagus and finely puree everything with a hand blender.
6. Squeeze the lemon. Stir the soy cream into the soup, season with salt, pepper, and a little lemon juice.
7. Heat the milk, a pinch of salt, and truffle oil (to approx. 60 ° C), do not let it boil! Whip the milk until frothy, e.g. with a hand blender, small whisk, or an electric milk frother. (The best results are achieved with low-fat long-life milk). Pour the soup into glasses or glass cups, distribute the milk foam on top. Serve immediately.

Nutritional values:

Calories 197 kcal (9%), Protein 10 g (10%), Fat 14 g (12%), Carb 6 g (4%), fibbers 2 g (7%)

46. Potato salad with asparagus

Cooking time: 30mins, total time 60mins, serving 4

Ingredients:

- 500 g mainly waxy potatoes
- salt
- 500 g green asparagus
- 5 tomatoes
- 1 handful chervil
- 200 ml vegetable broth
- 2 tbsp rapeseed oil
- 4 tbsp vinegar
- pepper
- 4 large lettuce leaves for garnish

Preparation steps:

1. Wash the potatoes thoroughly and cook them for about 20 minutes in salted water.
2. In the meantime, wash the asparagus, peel, and cut off the hard ends of the lower third. Cut the sticks into pieces diagonally, approx. Length: 3 cm. Cook for approximately 8 minutes in boiling salted water, then drain, rinse in cold water and drain.
3. The tomatoes are washed, the stalk is removed, and cut into wedges. Rinse the chervil and shake it dry, then finely chop it. Put aside about 4 stalks for garnish.
4. Drain the potatoes when the cooking time is over, rinse them, and peel them while they are still hot. Cut the potatoes into slices and pour over them with the hot stock. Mix in the tomatoes, asparagus, and chervil. Add oil and vinegar to the salad, salt, pepper, and season to taste.
5. Wash the leaves of the lettuce, shake them dry, and spread them over the bowls. Arrange the asparagus on top with the potato salad. Add the chervil to the garnish and serve.

Nutritional values:

Calories 178 kcal (8%), Protein 6 g (6%), Fat 5 g (4%), Carbohydrates 25 g (17%), added sugar 0 g (0%), fibbers 4.9 g (16%)

47. Chicken and asparagus salad with watercress

Preparation time 40mins, total time 50mins, serving 4

Ingredients:

- 100 g spring onions (0.5 bunch)
- 200 g cherry tomatoes
- 100 g green asparagus
- 600 g chicken breast fillet (4 chicken breast fillets)
- salt
- pepper
- 1 small lime
- 1 clove of garlic
- 6 tbsp honey
- 1 tbsp grainy mustard
- 5 tbsp olive oil
- 100 g watercress

Preparation steps:

1. Clean the spring onions and wash them and cut into thin rings. Wash the tomatoes and quarter. The woody ends of the asparagus are cut off. Wash and dry the asparagus. Halve the sticks and cut them into thin slices with a peeler in the half lengthways.
2. Wash the chicken fillets, pat dry with kitchen paper, and cut into strips. Season with salt and pepper. For the dressing, cut the lime in half and squeeze out the juice. Peel and dice the garlic. Mix with honey, mustard, 3 tablespoons of lime juice, and 3 tablespoons of oil. Season with salt and pepper. Heat the remaining oil in a large non-stick pan and stir-fry the meat for about 5 minutes over high heat.
3. Put the chicken, spring onions, tomatoes, and asparagus in a bowl. Mix in the dressing and let the salad steep for about 10 minutes.
4. In the meantime, wash the watercress and shake dry. Pluck the leaves, coarsely chop as desired, and distribute on plates or bowls. Season the chicken salad with salt and pepper and serve on the cress.

Nutritional values:

Calories 368 kcal (18%), Protein 37 g (38%), Fat 14 g (12%), Carbohydrates 22 g (15%), added sugar 17 g (68%), fibbers 2 g (7%)

48. Chicken and zucchini salad with nuts

Preparation time 30mins, total time 30mins, serving 4

Ingredients:

- 3 zucchinis
- 500 g chicken breast fillet
- salt
- pepper
- 4 tbsp olive oil
- ½ fret mint
- ½ lemon
- 80 g pecans

Preparation steps:

1. The zucchini must be washed and cleaned and cut into thin slices. Season with salt and pepper, rinse the chicken fillet under cold water, and pat dry.
2. In a pan, heat 2 tablespoons of oil. Fry the chicken in it for approximately 10 minutes over medium heat until golden brown. Reduce the heat and let the fillets of the chicken breast cook.

3. In another pan, heat the remaining oil. Sauté slices of zucchini in it for about 4 minutes over medium heat.
4. Wash the mint, shake the dry leaves, and pluck them. Squeeze the lemons in half.
5. Remove the chicken from the mixing bowl, drain it on kitchen paper and cut it into thin slices. Chop the nuts roughly and mix well with the zucchini, chicken, mint, and lemon juice. Use salt and pepper to season and arrange in bowls.

Nutritional values:

Calories 399 kcal (19%), Protein 36 g (37%), Fat 26 g (22%), Carbohydrates 6 g (4%), added sugar 0 g (0%), fibbers 4.1 g (14%)

49. Veal kidneys

Cooking time: 30mins, serving 4

Ingredients:

- 1 veal kidney 500 g
- Milk for inserting the kidney
- 1 onion 60 g
- 1 clove of garlic
- 2 tbsp olive oil
- 1 pinch sugar
- 150 ml dry sherry
- 50 g whipped cream
- 1 fresh bay leaf
- Salt
- Pepper from the mill
- 1 tbsp finely chopped tarragon

Preparation steps:

1. Halve the kidney of the veal longitudinally, parry, rinse well and cover for about 45 minutes with milk, then remove, pat dry, and cut into bite-sized pieces.
2. Peel the onion and garlic cloves, dice the onion coarsely and dice the garlic finely. Heat the oil in a pan, fry the kidney pieces in it quickly, remove them and keep warm.
3. Sweat the onions and garlic until translucent in the frying fat, sprinkle with the sugar, deglaze with sherry, put in the bay leaf, and cook for 5 minutes. Season with salt and pepper, remove the bay leaf, and remove the sauce from the stove. Stir in the cream and half of the tarragon, add the juice and kidneys and warm them up carefully (it should not boil anymore). Arrange the kidneys in a preheated bowl and serve the remaining tarragon sprinkled with it.

Nutritional values per serving (100 g):

Calories/Energy: 99 Kcal, Protein: 15.76 g (68.2%), Carbs: 0.85 g (3.3%), Fats: 3,12 g (28.5%), Sodium: 178 mg, Calcium: 11 mg, Phosphorous: 241 mg, Potassium: 272 mg

50. Zucchini risotto with kidneys

Cooking time 30mins, total time 3hrs, serving 4

Ingredients:

- 200 g pig kidney
- 1 shallot
- 2 tbsp oil
- 1 tbsp butter
- 7 sage leaves
- 3 tbsp sherry
- salt
- pepper from the grinder

For the risotto

- 700 ml vegetable broth (finished product)
- 1 onion
- 1 clove of garlic
- 80 g butter
- 250 g risotto rice
- 125 ml white wine
- salt
- pepper
- 1 zucchini
- 1 tbsp olive oil

Preparation steps:

1. Brush the kidneys, rinse and cover with water for about 2 hours.
2. For the risotto, bring the vegetable stock to the boil. Peel and dice the onion and garlic. Heat 40 g butter in a saucepan. Steam the onion, garlic, and rice until translucent. Deglaze with white wine. Gradually pour in the broth while stirring so that the rice is always covered. As soon as it has absorbed the liquid, pour in the broth again (this takes about 20-25 minutes).

3. Stir in the remaining butter in pieces and season with salt and pepper. Cover and let steep a little. Rinse, clean, and cut zucchini into pieces. Heat olive oil. Fry the zucchini in it for 3-4 minutes, season with salt and pepper, and mix with the risotto.
4. Pat the kidneys dry and cut into smaller pieces. Peel and dice shallot. Heat the oil and butter. Fry the kidneys in it for 12-15 minutes, adding the shallot cubes and the sage leaves. Deglaze with sherry, season with salt and pepper. Serve the risotto with the kidneys.

Nutritional values:

Calories/Energy: 101 Kcal, Lipids: 3 g, Carbs: 17 g, Protein: 2 g, Water: 77 g

51. Protein-free bucatini with broccoli

Serving: 1 - 4

Ingredients:

- 300 grams of bucatini ((or spaghetti) protein-free
- A pinch of salt
- (FOR THE DRESSING)
- 400 gr of broccoli
- 3 tablespoons of extra virgin olive oil
- 1 clove of garlic
- 4 anchovies in oil
- 10 gr of pine nuts
- 2 tablespoons of grated Parmesan cheese
- 2 tablespoons of grated pecorino Romano (an Italian cheese)
- 1 chili

Preparation:

1. Clean the broccoli by dividing the florets, wash them, and put them in a pot containing 4 litres of lightly boiling salted water. After 6-7 minutes they will be cooked, so drain them.
2. In a large pan, which must also contain the pasta, brown the garlic clove with the oil and anchovies. When it is golden, remove the garlic and add the chili, pine nuts, and broccoli. Allow to flavour by stirring.
3. Separately, cook the bucatini (or spaghetti) in 3 litres of slightly salted boiling water. Drain them al dente and cook them in the broccoli pan. Finally, season them with the grated Parmesan and pecorino. Serve immediately.

The use of protein-free paste must be prescribed by the nephrologist.

Nutritional values:

Protein: 8 g, Calories: 398 kcal, Potassium 8 *, Medium Phosphorus, Lipids: 12 g, Cholesterol: 9 mg

52. Protein-free spaghetti carbonara

Serving: 1 – 4

Ingredients:

- 300 gr of protein-free spaghetti
- A pinch of salt
- (FOR THE SEASONING)
- 150 gr of "guanciale"
- 3 egg yolks
- 80 gr of pecorino Romano

Preparation:

1. Boil 3 litres of water, add salt (a little) and throw in the spaghetti that you will cook "to the tooth".
2. Meantime: slowly brown the bacon that you have cut into thin strips in a small pan, no seasoning of any kind is needed because the melted fat of the bacon will be more than enough for seasoning; mix the beaten egg yolks with half of the grated cheese in a heated serving dish and dilute everything with a little pasta water.
3. When the spaghetti is cooked, transfer them to a serving dish, possibly without draining them but taking them from the pot with the special "take pasta" tongs so that they remain sufficiently moist and do not stick, season them quickly by pouring the bacon with its fat in the centre and the rest of the cheese. Serve immediately.

The use of protein-free paste must be prescribed by the nephrologist. Today, excellent protein-free pastas are on the market which do not require special cooking precautions compared to pastas produced with normal flours.

Nutritional values:

Protein: 11 g, Calories: 620 kcal, Low potassium 2 *, High Phosphorus, Lipids: 36 g, Cholesterol: 223 mg

53. Asparagus in salad with poached eggs

Serving: 1

Ingredients:

- 100 gr of asparagus already cleaned
- 1 fresh egg
- 1 tablespoon of white vinegar
- A pinch of salt
- (FOR THE DRESSING)
- 1 tablespoon of lemon juice
- 1 tablespoon of oil
- A modest pinch of salt
- A grind of black pepper

Preparation:

1. Carefully wash the asparagus in cold water, scrape the part of the stem with a small knife or a potato peeler and equalize them by breaking the final part with your hands, which will break by itself in the right place, to eliminate the hardest part.
2. Meanwhile, boil 3 litres of water in a pan large enough to hold the asparagus horizontally, throw in the asparagus and cook for 5-10 minutes. Change the first cooking water with another slightly salted and boiling water. Cook for another 5 minutes. When they are cooked according to your taste, drain them gently, let them dry on a cloth, and finally arrange them on the plate.
3. Separately, cook the poached egg proceeding as follows: in a large saucepan, half full of boiling water, add a pot of salt and vinegar; lower the heat, so that the water does not boil too strongly, then gently pour the egg that you have previously broken into a saucer. Using the skimmer, make sure that the egg white does not disperse. Cook slowly for 2-3 minutes and then, again with a slotted spoon, remove the egg from the saucepan, pass it in ice water to stop cooking, drain and dry it gently with kitchen paper or a towel.
4. Separately, beat the ingredients of the sauce, arrange the egg on the asparagus plate and serve with the sauce separately.

The potassium asterisks shown don't consider the double boiling of asparagus. Consider that the double boiling procedure reduces the values by about 1/3.

Nutritional values:

Protein: 11 g, Calories: 196 kcal, Potassium 7 *, Medium Phosphorus, Lipids: 15, Cholesterol: 223 mg

54. Protein-free bread dumplings

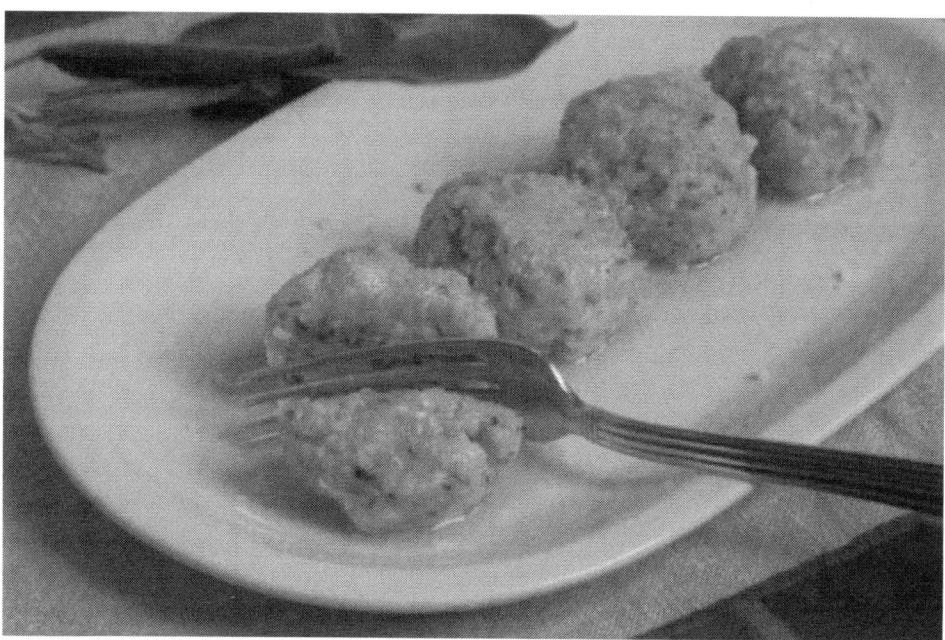

Serving: 1 - 4

Ingredients:

- (With the indicated doses you will get about 20 dumplings.)
- 3 stale protein-free rolls (about 200 g when fresh)
- 2 dl of protein-free milk
- 80 g smoked cooked ham (Prague ham)
- 15 g chopped parsley (about 2 tablespoons)
- 20 g of grated Parmesan cheese
- 1 egg
- 20 g of protein-free flour
- A grind of pepper
- A ground nutmeg
- A modest pinch of salt for the boiling water
- (FOR THE DRESSING)
- 40 g of butter
- 20 g of Parmesan cheese
- 2 sage leaves

Preparation:

1. Break the bread and put it in a bowl with the milk. Let it soak and then pulp it with a fork.

2. Add the chopped parsley, the grated Parmesan cheese, the coarsely chopped ham, the egg, and a sprinkle of pepper and nutmeg. Stir and add the flour a little at a time. You need to get a sufficiently dense dough so that you can form, with floured hands, gnocchi the size of an egg.
3. Boil the water in a large saucepan, add salt, and toss the gnocchi, adding them one at a time. Cook them for about 15 minutes, they will have to rise to the surface.
4. Drain them with a slotted spoon, place them in a heated serving dish, and season with the butter, which you have melted in a pan with the sage leaves, and the grated Parmesan. Serve them immediately.

*In the original recipe there would be speck, but I've replaced it with smoked cooked ham because it is too salty.**

Nutritional values:

Protein: 10 g, Calories: 332 kcal, Potassium 3 *, Medium Phosphorus, Lipids: 17 g, Cholesterol: 102 mg

55. Protein-free tagliatelle with courgettes and pistachios

Serving: 1 - 4

Ingredients:

- 250 g of protein-free tagliatelle (it is a pasta that yields a lot and therefore 250 g is enough for 4 people)
- 500 g of already cleaned zucchini
- 50 g vacuum-packed pistachios (already peeled and unsalted)
- 40 g of grated Parmesan cheese
- 1/2 lemon (a piece of peel in the pasta water and the juice of ½ lemon in the sauce)
- 1 bay leaf
- A bunch of mint (for flavour and garnish only)
- Salt (coarse for the pasta water and fine for the zucchini)
- 4 tablespoons of extra virgin olive oil

Preparation:

1. Slice the courgettes lengthwise, taking care to remove the inner part with the seeds, and arrange them in strips on the oven plate. Salt lightly and sprinkle them with very little oil. Put them in the oven at 200 ° for 8-10 minutes.
2. Coarsely chop both the cooked courgettes and the pistachios and place them in a bowl where you will dress the pasta.
3. Cook the pasta by putting a lemon peel and bay leaf in the cooking water.

4. Season in the tureen by adding the Parmesan, the mint leaves, the oil, and the juice of half a lemon.

There are excellent protein-free tagliatelle on the market that will allow you to prepare a tasty first course. I remind you that the use of protein-free products must always be prescribed by the doctor.

Nutritional values:

Protein: 8 g, Calories: 430 kcal, Potassium 9 *, Medium Phosphorus, Lipids: 20 g, Cholesterol: 9mg

56. Protein-free rice salad with Mediterranean pesto

Serving: 1 - 4

Ingredients:

- 200 g of low protein rice
- 150 g of tomatoes
- 80 g of courgettes (already cleaned)
- 1 tablespoon of apple cider vinegar
- A small pinch of salt for the rice cooking water
- A few drops of extra virgin olive oil to decorate
- (FOR THE MEDITERRANEAN PESTO)
- 40 g of pitted green olives
- 25 g of desalted capers
- 20 g of pine nuts
- 20 basil leaves
- 2 sprigs of fresh oregano
- A small fresh hot pepper, cleaned of seeds
- 1 clove of garlic
- 10 g of extra virgin olive oil

Preparation:

1. Prepare the Mediterranean pesto by pounding the ingredients in a mortar or blending.
2. Cook the low-protein rice, following the instructions on the package, and then shell it, allowing it to cool.
3. Clean the courgette, removing most of the inside to use the green part with little pulp, and cut it into cubes. Clean the tomato and cut it into wedges.
4. Season the cooled rice with pesto, courgette, tomato, and a tablespoon of apple cider vinegar.

Very tasty even without the addition of cheese: low in phosphorus and rich in taste!

Nutritional values:

Protein: 3 g, Calories: 247 kcal, Potassium 5 *, Low Phosphorus, Lipids: 7 g, Cholesterol: 0 mg

57. Protein-free Margherita pizza

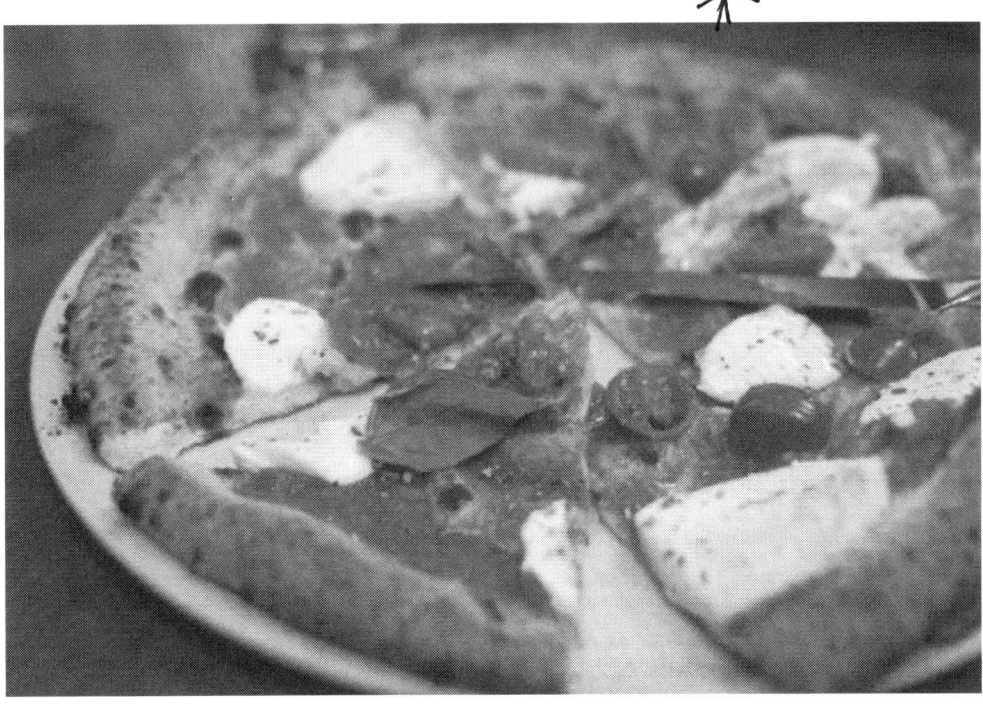

Serving: 1

Ingredients:

- 1 base for protein-free pizza of 150 g
- 60 g of tomato sauce
- 100 g of mozzarella
- 1 tablespoon of dried oregano
- 15 g of desalted capers
- 2 tablespoons of EVO oil

Preparation:

1. Place the pizza base on a plate covered with parchment paper.
2. Garnish with the tomato sauce, chopped mozzarella, capers, and dried oregano.
3. Drizzle with oil and bake following the instructions on the pizza base package.

There are some excellent protein-free pizza bases on the market. Here's how you can use them, naturally considering pizza as a single dish.

Nutritional values:

Protein: 21 g, Calories: 842 kcal, Potassium 10 *, Very high phosphorus, Lipids: 46 g, Cholesterol: 46 mg

58. Protein-free spaghetti "alla Norma"

Serving: 1 - 4

Ingredients:

- 300 g of protein-free spaghetti
- 50 g of chopped onion
- 300 g of eggplant
- 400 g of tomato pulp
- 1 clove of garlic
- 4 tablespoons of extra virgin olive oil
- 40 g of pecorino Romano
- Chili pepper
- A pinch of salt

Preparation:

1. Place Slice the eggplant into thin slices and pass them on a lightly greased plate or non-stick pan. Keep them aside.
2. Heat 3 tablespoons of olive oil in a large pan, add the clove of garlic and the finely sliced onion, brown, and add the tomato puree. Salt, add the chili, and cook for about 15 minutes. When cooked, if you don't like it, remove the garlic clove.
3. Meanwhile, cook the pasta in plenty of lightly salted water.
4. Once cooked, drain the pasta by collecting it from the pot with the special spaghetti collector tool and pass it, without draining it too much, into the pan with the sauce. Sauté for a minute adding the grilled aubergines.
5. Serve on hot plates and grate on each a few strands of pecorino Romano or salted ricotta cheese.

Nutritional values:

Protein: 5 g, Calories: 343 kcal, Potassium 10 *, Medium Phosphorus, Lipids: 16 g, Cholesterol: 9 mg

59. Protein-free penne with tuna and basil

Serving: 1 - 4

Ingredients:

- 400 g of protein-free penne
- 100 g of tuna in oil, already drained
- 1 clove of garlic
- 30 g of basil leaves
- 4 tablespoons of extra virgin olive oil
- 40 g of cherry tomatoes
- A pinch of salt

Preparation:

1. Clean the basil and blend the leaves with two tablespoons of oil and a very small pinch of salt.
2. Boil the pasta in salted water following the package instructions. Taste it to check the cooking and keep it al dente so that you can sauté it in a pan where, in the meantime, you have lightly fried the garlic with the remaining oil, add the well-drained tuna and the pureed basil. When the pasta is cooked to the right point, drain it, keeping a little cooking water, and pass it a couple of minutes in the pan with the tuna and basil.
3. In the end, with the fire off, add the cherry tomatoes and serve.

A pesto without cheese or pine nuts, but the taste of basil is always a good help in pasta sauces.

Nutritional values:

Protein: 7 g, Calories: 480 kcal, Potassium 3 *, Low Phosphorus, Lipids: 13 g, Cholesterol: 16 mg

60. Omelette with onions

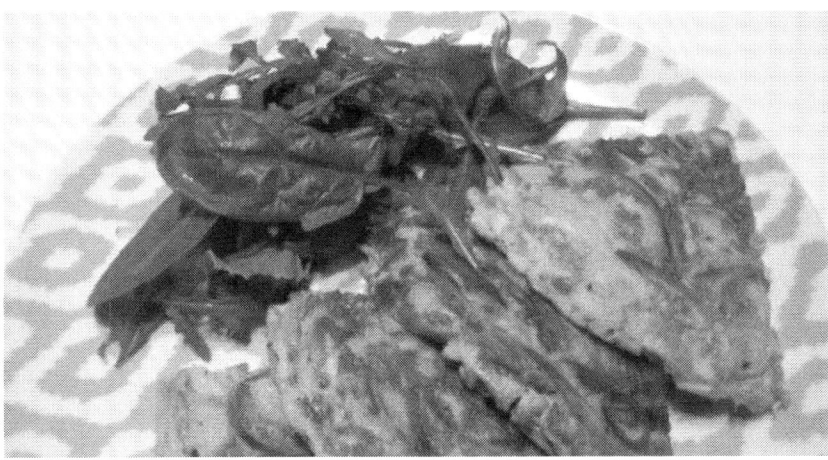

Serving: 1 - 4

Ingredients:

- 4 eggs
- 2 tablespoons of protein-free milk
- 150 g of onion already cleaned
- Two tablespoons of oil
- A pinch of salt
- A ground nutmeg
- A grind of pepper

Instructions:

1. Peel and wash the onions, then slice them and brown them in oil over moderate heat until they are slightly wilted.
2. Break the eggs into a bowl, add the milk, salt, pepper, and nutmeg and beat them with a fork, then add the browned onions.
3. Grease a non-stick pan and let it heat up, pour the egg and onion mixture into it and stir until it starts to thicken. Cover with a lid and let the omelette set completely on one side. At this point, turn it over with the lid and let it thicken on the other side as well.
4. Transfer the omelette to a serving dish and slice it.

Nutritional Information:

Protein: 8 g, Calories: 136 kcal, Potassium 3 *, Low Phosphorus, Lipids: 10 g, Cholesterol: 223 mg

61. Lentils with cotechino

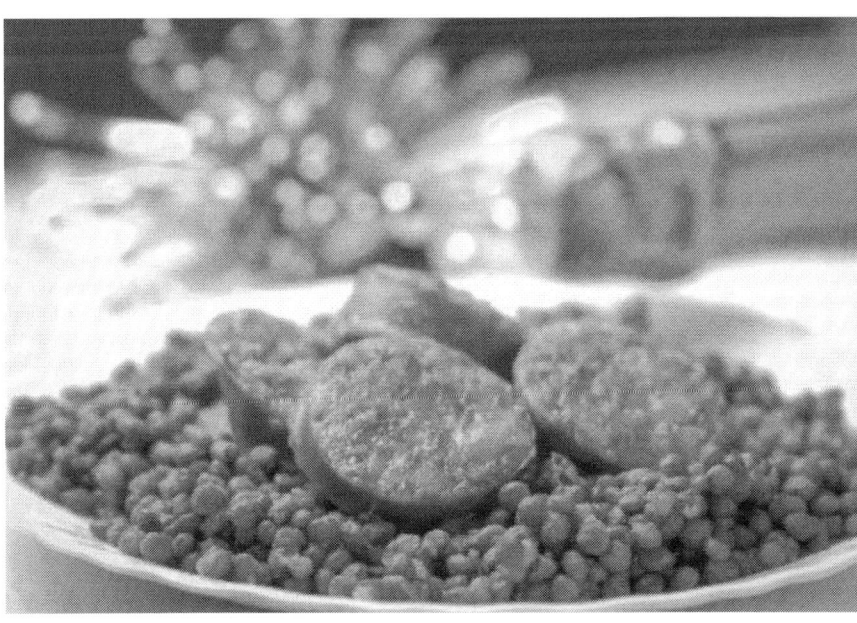

Serving: 6

Ingredients:

- 300 g of lentils
- 200 g of tomato pulp
- Extra virgin olive oil 40 g
- Garlic
- Parsley
- Salt
- Pepper
- Chilli to taste
- A precooked cotechino - about 500 g

Preparation:

1. Clean the lentils to remove any impurities and soak them; eliminate those that have surfaced. Leave them to soak for a few hours by changing the water: with this procedure, part of the potassium dissolves in the water. Then put them in a saucepan and cover with clean water. Bring to a boil and then replace the water with the same clean one. Salt as permitted.
2. Meanwhile, prepare the sauce: crush and chop the garlic and heat it in oil together with the chili if you like; add the tomato and cook for a few minutes; add the chopped parsley. Drain the lentils a little and add them to the saucepan, stir, let them take on flavour for 10 minutes.
3. While the lentils are cooking, boil the cotechino too, following the instructions on the package. Drain it, let it cool and cut it into slices. Put in the pan with the stewed lentils to flavour. Serve hot.

Lentil is characterized by a skin so thin that it does not need to be soaked before cooking; it has a high content of protein, iron, mineral salts, and fibbers. It is excellent to accompany cold cuts such as cotechino and zampone. The reported potassium value refers to raw foods; soaking and changing the cooking water reduce it. Sodium is the one contained in cotechino.

Nutritional values:

Water: 178 g, Protein: 29 g, Phosphorous: 325 mg, Potassium: 670 mg, Lipids: 34 g, Carbs: 28 g, Sodium: 642 mg, Calories: 531 kcal

62. Pizzoccheri

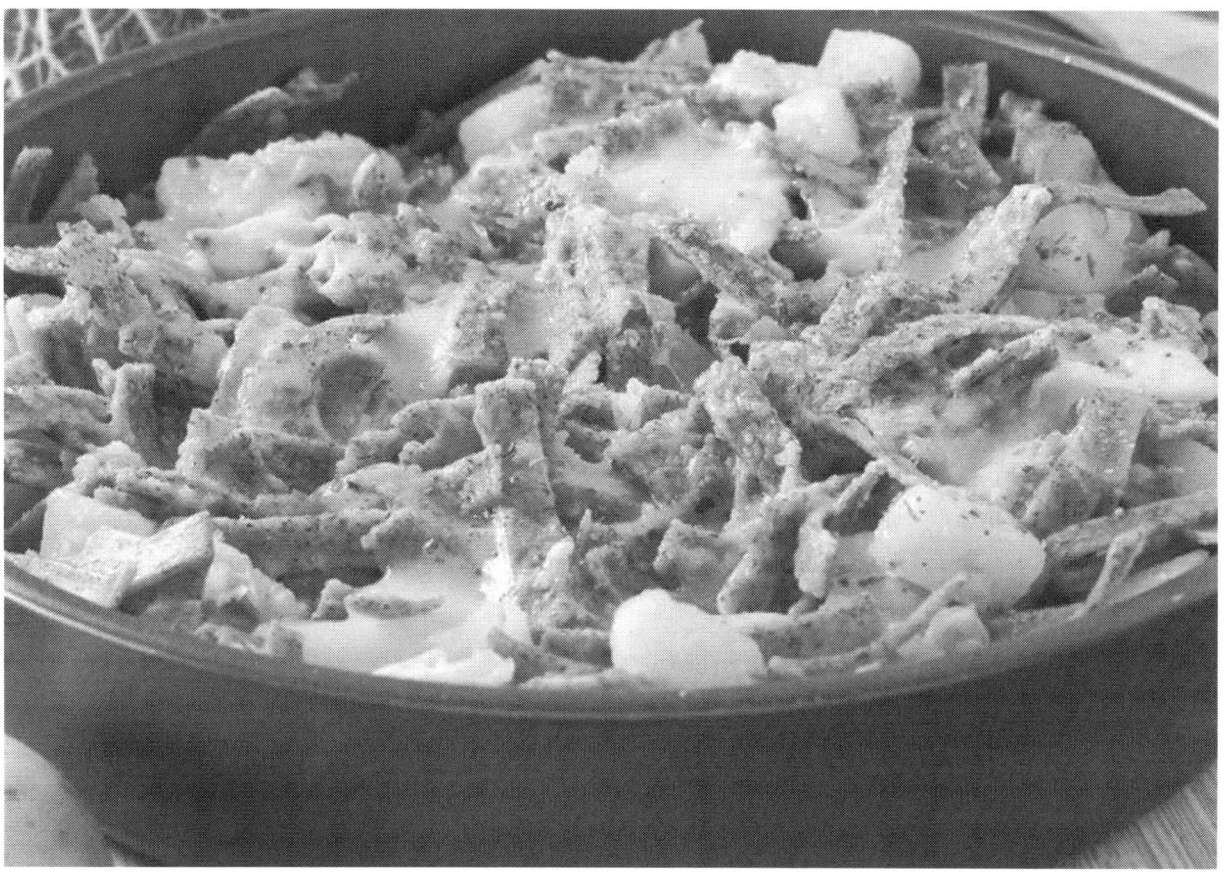

Serving: 6

Ingredients:

- Pizzoccheri 500 g
- Potatoes 500 g
- Chard 300 g
- Cabbage 400 g
- Fontina cheese 250 g
- Parmesan 50 g
- Butter 100 g
- Sage and garlic
- Salt if included in your diet

Preparation:

1. Put a large pot of salted water to boil. When it boils, add the diced potatoes, chard and cabbage cut into small pieces. Cook for 5 minutes. Then add the pizzoccheri and cook for 15 minutes.

2. Meanwhile, prepare the sauce in a large pan: peel the garlic, mash it and fry it with the butter and sage. Cut the fontina into small pieces.
3. When the pizzoccheri are cooked, drain them with a slotted spoon and put them to flavour in the butter. Add the cheeses and stir until they melt.

It is a dish to be consumed very rarely as it is rich in fat, in particular saturated fat. Be careful with this dish: it is rich in phosphorus and potassium. This serving provides half the daily amount of these nutrients for a person on dialysis!

Nutritional values:

Water: 287 g, Protein: 25 g, Phosphorous: 488 mg, Potassium: 954 mg, Lipids: 30 g, Carbs: 76 g, Sodium: 491 mg, Calories: 680 kcal

63. Butterflies with hake fillets and courgette flowers

Serving: 1 - 4

Ingredients:

- Hake fillets 240 g
- 1 level spoonful of flour
- Olives oil 10 g
- Courgette flowers 100 g
- Shallot
- Chili pepper
- Half a clove of garlic
- Mint and tarragon
- Basil
- Parsley
- 1 teaspoon of turmeric
- Semolina pasta 50 g

Preparation:

1. Heat the water for the pasta, salt it if allowed, and add a teaspoon of turmeric.
2. Meanwhile, prepare the dressing. Clean the courgette flowers by removing the pistil and cut them roughly; set aside.
3. Chop the shallot and the garlic clove; brown them in a large pan in olive oil adding the chili. Lightly flour the hake fillets, place them in the pan and cook over low heat for about 10-15 minutes, adding a little water from the pasta. Chop the fillets so they can cook better. Add the

chopped mint and tarragon. Remove the chili from the sauce and add the courgette flowers, mix gently (if it dries too much, add a little water from the pasta).

4. In the meantime, throw the pasta: I used the butterfly shape, but you choose the pasta you like best.
5. Drain the pasta al dente and pour it into the fish pan; add some chopped and whipped basil leaves. With the fire off, add the chopped parsley, a sprinkle of ground white pepper, 2 basil leaves to decorate and enjoy your meal.

This is a unique dish, excellent for those who do peritoneal dialysis because it is very rich in proteins. The water is calculated taking into consideration what the pasta absorbs during cooking.

Nutritional values:

Water: 400 g, Protein: 47 g, Phosphorous: 553 mg, Potassium: 1126 mg, Lipids: 12 g, Carbs: 60 g, Sodium: 178 mg, Calories: 525 kcal

64. Pasta and chickpeas

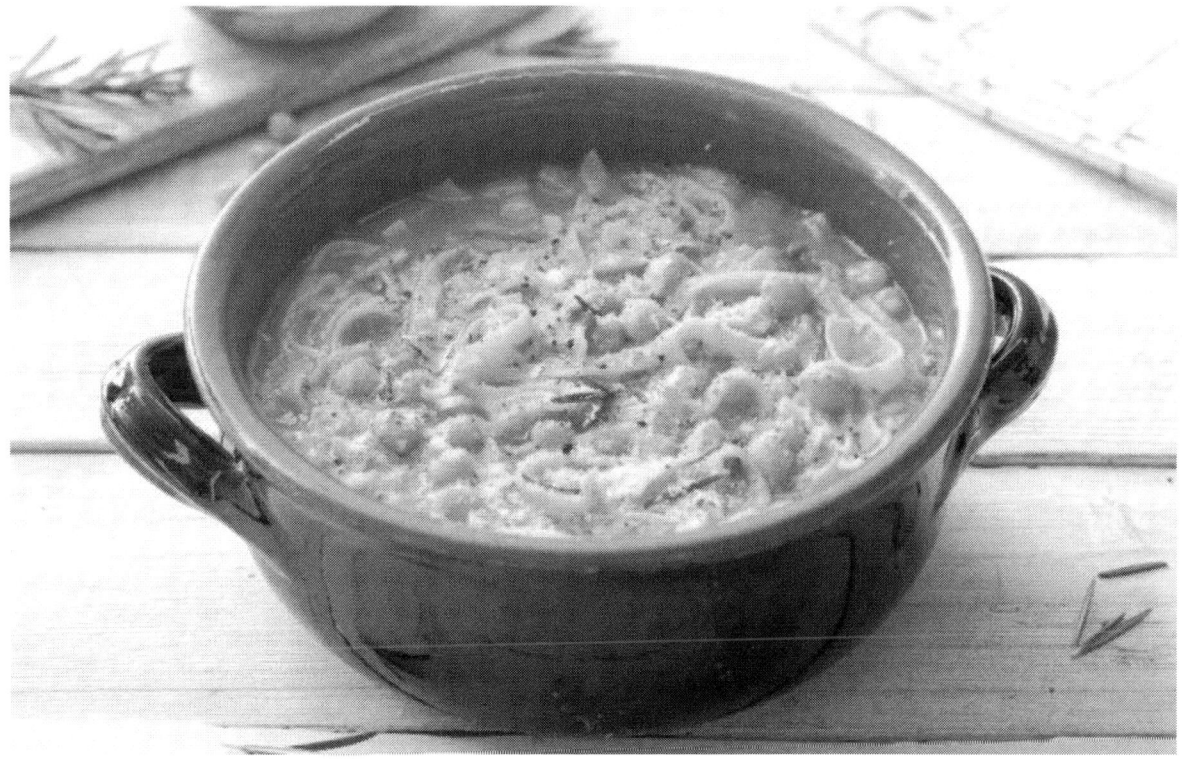

Serving: 4

Ingredients:

- Boiled chickpeas 2 boxes 480 g
- Potato 150 g
- Onion 50 g

- Celery 30 g
- Ripe tomato 100 g
- 1 clove of garlic
- 1 sprig of rosemary
- Extra virgin olive oil 50 g
- Semolina pasta 120 g

Preparation:

1. Peel the potato and cut it into pieces; coarsely chopped onion, tomato, and celery; put everything in a pot with 1 tablespoon of extra virgin olive oil, the clove of garlic, and the rosemary. Cover with water and cook until soft. Remove the rosemary and add one of the cans of chickpeas drained from the liquid. Cook for a few more minutes and then blend everything with an immersion blender.
2. Now add the other jar of chickpeas and add just enough water. Cook for another half hour and then add the short pasta. Bring to cooking. Before serving, add a nice spoonful of raw extra virgin olive oil (and black pepper if you like).
3. In summer it is excellent if prepared in advance and eaten warm.

Due to the reduced protein content this recipe is suitable for a conservative diet. The combination of legume proteins with those of cereals improves the protein quality. In dialysis, I recommend adding a small portion of a second dish.

Nutritional values:

Water: 350 g, Protein: 13 g, Phosphorous: 177 mg, Potassium: 515 mg, Lipids: 16 g, Carbs: 49 g, Sodium: 360 mg, Calories: 380 kcal

65. Pasta with sardines

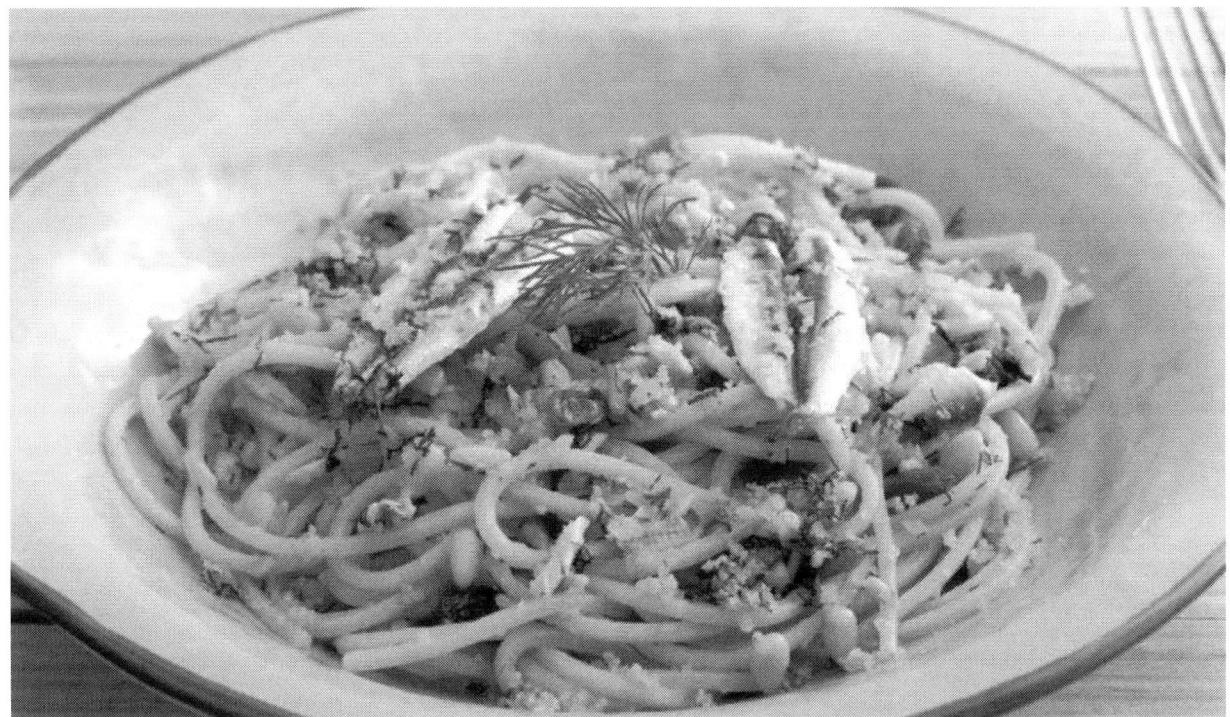

Serving: 4

Ingredients:

- Fresh sardines to clean 300 g
- 1 onion
- Garlic
- Pickled capers 20 g
- Eggplant 200 g
- Extra virgin olive oil 50 g
- Hot pepper
- Chopped parsley
- Pasta 320 g

Preparation:

1. Cook the pasta and while it is cooking, prepare: chopped onion that you will brown in oil with the garlic; add the drained capers, diced eggplant, chopped sardines. Cook over medium heat, stirring occasionally; add a little cooking water from the pasta to mix
2. The cooking time of the sauce is practically that of the pasta (10 minutes approx.). Add chili to taste.
3. Drain the pasta and pour it into the pan in which you prepared the sauce.

4. Turn off and add the chopped parsley. Stir well and serve immediately.

The sodium reported is that of food, without additions. The protein content makes this dish an excellent single dish for conservative therapy.

Nutritional values:

Water: 220 g, Protein: 21 g, Phosphorous: 273 mg, Potassium: 660 mg, Lipids: 15 g, Carbs: 70 g, Sodium: 132 mg, Calories: 481 kcal

66. Rice with baby octopus and radicchio

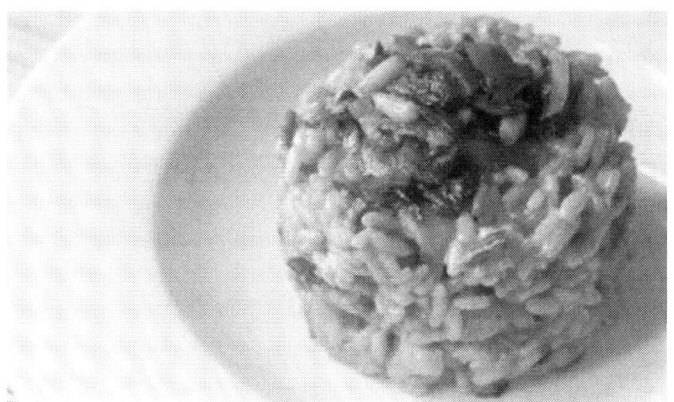

Serving: 1

Ingredients:

- Parboiled rice 50 g
- Red radicchio 70 g
- Leek 10 g
- 1 clove of garlic
- Red pepper
- Cleaned octopus 170 g
- Extra virgin olive oil 15 g
- A little white wine
- 1 teaspoon of turmeric
- A sprig of parsley
- Pepper

Preparation:

1. Clean, wash, and cut the radicchio into pieces. Bring a little water to the boil, add the rice and radicchio and let it boil for 10 minutes.
2. Meanwhile, brown the garlic and finely chopped leek in the oil. Shred the octopus, add it to the sauté and blend with the white wine.

3. Drain the radicchio and rice and add it to the baby octopus. Add the chili and turmeric dissolved in a little hot water. Bring the rice to cook while continuing to stir and adding hot water when needed, about another 10 minutes.
4. Turn off the heat, cover the pot and let the risotto rest for a few minutes.
5. Remove the chili pepper, plant, add the chopped parsley, and a sprinkle of ground pepper.

Single and unique dish for people on dialysis. For the calculation of the nutrients, I used octopus because the baby octopus are not listed in the composition tables. The water considered is also absorbed by the rice during cooking. It is a dish a little rich in phosphorus: you can boil the octopus separately to remove some of it.

Nutritional values:

Water: 301 g, Protein: 23 g, Phosphorous: 413 mg, Potassium: 827 mg, Lipids: 18 g, Carbs: 47 g, Sodium: 403 mg, Calories: 427 kcal

CHAPTER NINE: Soup and Stew Recipes

67. Chili con carne

Preparation time 30mins, total time 2hrs, serving 8

Ingredients:

- 1/2 cup onions
- 1 stick of celery
- 1/2 cup green bell peppers
- 675 grams of lean ground beef
- 450 grams of chopped canned tomatoes (low in salt)
- 1 tablespoon of canola oil
- 2 tablespoons of chili powder
- 1 1/2 cups of water

Preparation:

1. Chop the onion, celery, and paprika.
2. Fry the onions, celery, and peppers over medium heat until golden brown.
3. Add the minced meat, cut into small pieces and fry well.
4. Add the canned tomatoes to the minced meat, add the chili powder and water, reduce over low heat.
5. let simmer for some time.

Nutritional values:

Calories 190, Protein 20 g, Carbohydrates 5 g, Fat 10 g, Cholesterol 57 mg, Sodium 116 mg, Potassium 450 mg, Phosphorus 180 mg, Calcium 38 mg, Dietary fibbers 1.3 g

68. Creamy chicken soup with wild rice and asparagus

Serving 8

Ingredients:

- 160 g wild rice
- 950 ml chicken broth
- 3 cloves of garlic
- 80 g onions
- 130 g carrots
- 90 g asparagus, white

- 55 g butter, unsalted
- 65 g wheat flour, type 405
- 950 ml of water
- 120 ml Martini Extra Dry
- 280 g chicken, cooked
- 1/2 teaspoon thyme
- 1 bay leaf
- 1/4 teaspoon nutmeg
- 1/2 teaspoon salt
- Milled pepper to taste
- 950 ml almond milk, unsweetened

Preparation:

1. For 30 minutes, soak the wild rice in hot water. Pouring away.
2. Put the rice into a pan with the chicken stock. Bring it slowly to a boil, then reduce the heat. Simmer for around 45 minutes with the lid closed.
3. Remove the pan from the heat and, with the lid closed, let the rice steep for another 15 minutes. Let it cool.
4. Chop the garlic finely. Cut the onion, carrots, and asparagus into cubes.
5. In a Dutch oven or large saucepan, melt the butter and sweat it with the garlic and onion. Add the carrots, spices, and herbs. Until everything is soft, continue cooking.
6. Add the flour and reduce it for about 10 minutes over low heat. Stir regularly.
7. Pour the water and the martini into it. With a whisk, stir vigorously.
8. Slice the chicken into small chunks. In the pot, put the meat and asparagus. Pour in the almond milk gradually. For 20 minutes, let it simmer.
9. Fold the wild rice in it and serve.

Nutritional value:

Calories 295, Protein 21 g, Carbohydrates 28 g, Fat 11 g, Cholesterol 45 mg, Sodium 385 mg, Potassium 527 mg, Phosphorus 252 mg, Calcium 183 mg, Dietary fibbers 3.3 g

69. Cold cucumber soup

Servings: 4 servings

Ingredients:

- 2 medium-sized cucumbers (600 g)
- 50 g shallots
- 1 spring onion (15 g)

- 5 g fresh mint
- 2 teaspoons of fresh dill
- 2 teaspoons of lemon juice
- 160 ml of water
- 120ml cream-milk mixture
- 65 g sour cream
- 1/2 teaspoon pepper
- 1/4 teaspoon salt
- Fresh dill sprigs for garnish (optional)

Preparation:

- Peel and core the cucumber. Finely chop the onions and mint. Chop up the dill.
- Put all ingredients in the mixer and puree.
- Place covered in the fridge.
- Garnish the soup with fresh sprigs of dill as desired.

Nutritional value:

78 calories, 2 g white eggs, 6 g carbohydrates, 5 g fat, 12 mg cholesterol, 128 mg sodium, 256 mg potassium, 64 mg phosphorus, 60 mg calcium, 1.0 g dietary fibber

70. Pumpkin and walnut puree

Preparation time 10mins, total time 10mins, serving 6

Ingredients:

- 100 g walnuts, without shell
- 300 g pumpkin
- 30 ml of milk
- 600 ml of water

Preparation:

1. Peel the walnuts and pound them with the mortar.
2. Peel the pumpkin and cut into pieces. Place the pumpkin pieces in a plastic bag and place it in the microwave over a high temperature for five minutes.
3. Put the water with the pumpkin and walnuts in the blender and puree.
4. Put everything in a saucepan and cook until mushy over low heat.
5. Slowly pour in the milk and stir.

Nutrients per serving:

Calories 53, White eggs 2 g, Carbohydrates 4 g, Fat 4 g, Cholesterol 1 mg, Sodium 167 mg, Potassium 201 mg, Calcium 23 mg, Phosphorus 59 mg, Dietary fibber 1.2 g

71. Andean soup

Serving 4

Ingredients:

- 1 medium-headed white onion
- 1 stalk of long onion (green)
- 3 garlic cloves
- 1/4-pound low-fat mozzarella cheese
- 4 medium potatoes
- 1/2 litre low sodium chicken broth
- 1/2 litre of water
- 2 ounces milk
- 1 branch of coriander
- 4 eggs

Preparation:

1. Finely chop the onions and cilantro. Macerate the garlic.
2. Cut the cheese into small pieces.
3. Peel and dice the potatoes. Cover the potatoes completely with water and bring to a boil. Drain and repeat the process. Separate the potatoes.
4. Bring the broth to a boil with the onions and garlic.
5. Stir in the potatoes, milk, and cheese.
6. When the cheese is melted add the coriander.
7. When turning off the heat, add 4 eggs to the soup one by one, taking care not to break them.

Nutrients per serving:

Calories 288, Protein 19 g, Carbohydrates 27 g, Fat 14 g, Cholesterol 205 mg, Sodium 350 mg, Potassium 524 mg, Phosphorus 369 mg, Calcium 276 mg, fibbers 1.6 g

72. Bean and pepper soup with coriander

Preparation time 30mins, total time 50mins, serving 4

Ingredients:

- 1 onion
- 2 garlic cloves
- 2 tbsp. olive oil
- 2 red peppers
- 800 ml vegetable broth
- salt
- cayenne pepper
- Tabasco
- curry powder
- 2 cans kidney beans á 240 g
- 200 ml whipped cream at least 30% fat content
- 1 coriander

Preparation steps:

1. Peel the onion and garlic, diced finely, and sauté in a saucepan with hot oil until translucent. Wash the bell peppers, cut in half, core, dice, and add. Sweat briefly and deglaze with the broth. Season with salt, cayenne pepper, curry, and Tabasco and simmer over medium heat for 10 minutes.
2. Pour the beans over a sieve, rinse with cold water and drain well. Stir the cream with the beans into the soup and simmer for another 4 minutes. Wash the coriander, shake dry, pluck the leaves off, and roughly chop.
3. Season the soup to taste, season again if necessary, pour into preheated bowls, and serve sprinkled with the coriander. Serve with a fresh baguette if you like.

Nutritional values:

Calories 357 kcal (17%), Protein 14 g (14%), Fat 22 g (19%), Carbohydrates 26 g (17%), added sugar 0 g (0%), fibbers 14.1 g (47%)

73. Bean and ham soup with bread

Cooking time: 1h, serving 4

Ingredients:

- 1 onion
- 2 garlic cloves
- 250 g sweet potatoes
- 1 red chili pepper
- 100 g ham
- 2 tbsp vegetable oil
- 1 l meat soup
- 100 g dried kidney beans
- 100 g dried white lima bean
- 250 g pizza tomatoes
- 2 tbsp tomato paste
- Tabasco
- Salt
- Pepper from the mill
- 4 rye rolls

Preparation steps:

1. Mix the beans, pour water over them, and leave to soak overnight. The next day, peel and finely chop the onion and garlic. Wash the chili pepper, slit lengthways, core, and chop very finely. Finely dice the ham. Peel the sweet potato and cut into pieces of equal size.
2. Heat the oil in a large saucepan, sauté the onions and garlic until translucent. Fry the ham and tomato paste in it, season with salt and pepper. Add the chili and sweet potatoes and fry briefly. Add the stock and beans (without soaking water), mash the tomatoes with a fork, add to the beans.
3. Season with Tabasco and cover and simmer over low heat for about 30-40 minutes. If necessary, add some more broth and season the bean soup to taste. Serve with the rye rolls.

Nutritional values per serving:

Calories/Energy: 181 Kcal, Carbs: 33.5 g (Sugars: 7.8 g) (67.7%), Protein: 10.3 g (20.8%), Lipids: 2.5 g (11.6%), Fibbers: 9.3 g, Cholesterol: 4.9 mg, Water: 195.8 g, Sodium: 0.5 g, Calcium: 93.1 mg, Phosphorous: 31.9 mg, Potassium: 387.1 mg

74. Hearty vegetable soup with bacon

Cooking time: 1 h 15 min, total time 13 h 15 min, serving 4

Ingredients:

- 250 g dried kidney beans
- 150 g smoked bacon
- 1 large onion
- 2 garlic cloves
- 3 tomatoes
- 1 small savoy cabbage
- 4 potatoes
- 2 tbsp olive oil
- 1 ½ l meat soup
- salt
- pepper from the mill

Preparation steps:

1. Soak the dried beans in plenty of cold water overnight.
2. The next day, drain the beans and cook them halfway through in fresh cold water for about 30–40 minutes.
3. In the meantime, dice the bacon. Peel onion and garlic and chop finely. Scald the tomatoes with boiling water for a few seconds, rinse, peel, quarter, core, and chop.
4. Clean and wash the cabbage, quarter lengthways, cut off the stalk, and cut the quarters crosswise into strips. Peel the potatoes and cut into bite-sized pieces.
5. Heat the olive oil in a large saucepan and briefly brown the onions, garlic cloves, and bacon. Pour the meat stock. Add tomatoes, savoy cabbage strips, and potatoes. Drain the beans and stir into the stock under the vegetables. Salt and pepper and let simmer on low heat for about 30 minutes.

Nutritional values:

Calories 567 kcal (27%), Protein 17 g (17%), Fat 40 g (34%), Carbohydrates 36 g (24%), added sugar 0 g (0%), fibbers 15.1 g (50%)

75. Mexican-style chicken and vegetable soup

Preparation: 40 min, total time 3 h 10 min, serving 4

Ingredients:

- 1 soup chicken
- 3 onions
- 2 carrots
- 150 g celery root
- 1 bay leaf
- 2 cloves
- 1 tsp peppercorns
- 1 tbsp rapeseed oil
- 2 green peppers
- 1 red chili pepper
- 6 tomatoes
- 1 can of kidney beans
- 1 can corn
- salt
- pepper

Preparation steps:

1. Wash the chicken soup and cover it with cold water in a saucepan that is large enough. Simmer. Boil. Meanwhile, peel 2 onions, carrots, and celery, and roughly dice them. Add the bay leaves, cloves, and peppercorns to the chicken and cook for about 2 hours, just below the boiling point, over medium heat. If necessary, skim off the foam occasionally and add water.
2. Take the chicken out of the soup and let it cool. Pour the stock through a sieve and measure 1 litre (otherwise use the remainder). Peel the chicken and the skin is removed. Have the meat cut into strips.
3. Peel the remaining onion and dice it. In a saucepan, sweat in hot oil until it is translucent. Pour the stock into it and bring it to a boil. In the meantime, wash, cut in half, clean and dice the peppers and chili. Scald the hot-water tomatoes, rinse, peel, quarter, core, and dice. Drain the beans and maize and add bell pepper, chili, tomatoes, and chicken to the soup.
4. For about 15 minutes, let everything simmer together. Season with pepper and salt and serve.

Nutritional values:

Calories/Energy: 69 Kcal, Protein: 5.13 g, Carbs: 7.87 g, Lipids: 2.01 g, Sodium: 347 mg, Calcium: 11 mg, Potassium: 153 mg, Phosphorous: 44 mg

76. Mexican bean soup

Cooking time 25mins, total time 45mins, serving 4

Ingredients:

- 4 tomatoes
- 150 g green beans
- 1 onion
- 1 clove of garlic
- 1 red chili pepper
- 2 tbsp olive oil
- 2 tbsp tomato paste
- 1 tsp paprika noble sweet
- 1 tsp ground cumin
- 1 tsp ground coriander
- 1 l vegetable broth
- 240 g kidney beans (can; drained weight)
- 240 g white beans (can; drained weight)
- Salt
- Pepper
- Coriander greens for garnish

Preparation steps:

1. Scald, quench, peel, remove the stalk and roughly chop the tomatoes with hot water. Wash the green beans, clean them, and cut them into small pieces. Peel and chop the onion and garlic finely. Wash and clean the chili, remove the seeds and, if desired, finely chop it.
2. In a saucepan, heat the oil and fry the onion, garlic, and chili in it. Sauté the tomato paste and add paprika, cumin, and cilantro to the mixture. Put the broth in and bring it to a boil. Add the green beans and tomatoes and simmer over low heat for about 10 minutes. The kidney and white beans are drained, washed, and added. Let it simmer for an additional 5 minutes. Serve in bowls with coriander leaves and season with salt and pepper.

Nutritional values:

Calories 205 kcal (10%), Protein 13 g (13%), Fat 6 g (5%), Carbohydrates 23 g (15%), added sugar 0 g (0%), fibbers 12.8 g (43%)

77. Bean and potato stew

Serving 4

Ingredients:

- 1 onion
- 1 clove of garlic
- 300 g waxy potatoes
- 350 g white broad bean jar
- 350 g kidney beans can
- 120 g bacon slices
- 800 ml vegetable broth
- 300 g passed tomatoes
- 1 tsp dried marjoram
- salt
- pepper from the mill
- parsley for garnish

Preparation steps:

1. Peel and slice the onion, garlic, and potatoes into small cubes. Rinse a sieve with the beans and drain well.
2. Cut half the bacon into thin strips and put them in a casserole dish. Add the onion, garlic and potatoes, sweat briefly, and let the stock deglaze. Stir the tomatoes in and simmer for about 10 minutes over medium heat. Season with salt, pepper, and simmer gently for another 5-10 minutes. Then add the beans and marjoram. Season to taste and serve with parsley and garnish.
3. In a pan, fry the rest of the bacon until crispy, drain on paper towels and serve with the stew.

Nutritional values:

Calories 380 kcal (18%), Protein 15 g (15%), Fat 20 g (17%), Carbohydrates 33 g (22%), added sugar 0 g (0%), fibbers 12 g (40%)

78. Clear soup with vegetables

Preparation time 20mins, total time 40mins, serving 4

Ingredients:

- 200 g waxy potatoes
- 2 poles celery
- 4 spring onions
- 1 onion
- 2 garlic cloves
- 2 yellow peppers
- 2 tbsp olive oil
- 1 tbsp tomato paste
- 1 l vegetable broth
- 400 g kidney beans can
- 2 fresh bay leaves
- salt
- pepper

Preparation steps:

1. Peel and dice the potatoes, clean and wash the celery and spring onions and cut into rings. Peel and chop the onion and garlic. Clean the peppers, cut in half, remove the seeds and white skins, wash and cut into thin strips.
2. Heat the oil in a hot saucepan and sauté the vegetables for 2-3 minutes over medium heat. Fry the tomato paste briefly, then pour in the stock and bring to the boil once. In the meantime, drain the beans and wash them. Add to the clear soup together with the bay leaf. Season with salt and pepper and simmer over low heat for about 15 minutes.
3. Season the soup again to taste and serve in bowls.

Nutritional values:

Calories 227 kcal (11%), Protein 12 g (12%), Fat 6 g (5%), Carbohydrates 30 g (20%), added sugar 0 g (0%), fibbers 13.5 g (45%)

79. Bean stew with beef fillet

Cooking time 25mins, serving 4

Ingredients:

- 50 g kidney beans (can; drained weight)
- 50 g small white beans (can; drained weight)
- ½ onion
- 1 small clove of garlic
- ½ red pepper
- 2 tsp olive oil
- 1 branch thyme
- 1 bay leaf
- 200 chunky tomatoes (can)
- salt
- pepper
- cayenne pepper
- ¼ tsp ground coriander
- 150 g beef fillet
- 1 stem basil

Preparation steps:

1. In a sieve, rinse both types of beans and let them drain. Peel the garlic and onion and cut them into fine cubes. Wash, clean, core, and slice the peppers.
2. In a casserole, heat one teaspoon of oil. Sauté the onion and garlic in it over medium heat for 2 minutes. Wash the thyme and the bay leaves and add the beans and tomatoes to the saucepan, season with salt, pepper, cayenne pepper, and coriander and cook for about 15-17 minutes over medium heat, stirring occasionally.
3. Rinse the beef, pat dry and cut into thin strips about 20 minutes before cooking time ends. In a pan, heat the remaining oil. For 2-3 minutes, fry the beef fillet strips over high heat. With salt and pepper, season.
4. Wash the basil, shake it dry, and finely chop it. Top the bean stew with the meat and basil.

Nutritional values:

Calories 393 kcal (19%), Protein 40 g (41%), Fat 17 g (15%), Carbohydrates 19 g (13%), added sugar 0 g (0%), fibbers 10.4 g (35%)

80. Nutmeg pumpkin soup with kidney beans

Serving 4

Ingredients:

- 1 kg nutmeg pumpkin
- 2 dice vegetable broth
- 1 tbsp olive oil
- 1 lemon
- 400 g kidney beans (1 can, drained weight)
- 2 stems parsley
- pepper
- salt

Preparation steps:

1. The pumpkin is cleaned and peeled, the core removed and the pulp cut into cubes. In a saucepan, put the pumpkin cubes in. To just cover the pumpkin, add sufficient water. Bring it to a boil and add 2 cubes of stock. Cook for 20 minutes over medium heat until the pumpkin is tender.
2. Cut the lemon in half and squeeze the juice out. Drain the kidney beans in a colander, rinse and drain with hot water. Wash the parsley, shake it dry and, except for a few leaves, chop finely.
3. Add the oil to the pumpkin at the end of the cooking time and finely puree it all with a hand blender. Season with lemon juice, pepper, and a little salt if necessary. Distribute the beans and pour hot soup over them on 4 soup plates. Serve with parsley, sprinkled.

Nutritional values:

Calories 197 kcal (9%), Protein 12 g (12%), Fat 4 g (3%), Carbohydrates 27 g (18%), added sugar 0 g (0%), fibbers 15 g (50%)

81. Zucchini soup

Ingredients for 4 persons:

- 2 large zucchinis
- 1 onion
- 2 potatoes
- 2 carrots
- 1 tbsp (sesame oil, coconut fat, refined rapeseed or olive oil) frying oil
- 500 ml vegetable broth
- 100 g (natural, 15% fat in dry matter) cream cheese

- ½ bunch of parsley
- Salt and pepper

Preparation:

1. Wash and dice the zucchini. Peel the onion, potatoes, and carrots, then dice them.
2. Heat the oil in a pot. Sweat the onion cubes in it until they are golden yellow. Add the rest of the vegetables and fry briefly. Deglaze with the vegetable stock and simmer for about 10 minutes. When the vegetables are soft, puree the soup.
3. Stir the cream cheese into the warm soup and season with salt and pepper. Wash and finely chop the parsley and serve on top of the soup.

Nutritional values:

Calories/Energy: 36.04 Kcal, Carbs: 4.07 g (39.8%), Lipids: 1.68 g (37%), Protein: 2.38 g (23.3%)

82. Quick pea soup

Total time 20mins, preparation 5mins, serving 3

Ingredients:

- 300 g Potatoes
- 1 onion
- 1 toe garlic
- 30 g butter
- 200 g cream
- 1 Bay leaf
- 400 g frozen peas
- Salt
- Pepper
- Nutmeg
- Cumin
- As required: smoked salmon

Preparation:

1. Peel the potatoes, onion, and garlic and cut into cubes. Melt the butter in a saucepan and sauté potatoes, onions, and garlic in it.
2. Deglaze with cream, fill the cup twice with water and add this as well. Season with salt, pepper, freshly grated nutmeg, and cumin.

3. Add the bay leaf and cook everything until the potatoes are done. Take out the bay leaf and add the peas. Bring to the boil again and then puree with a hand blender. If the soup is still too thick, add 1 more shot of water.
4. Season again to taste and serve. Add smoked salmon strips to the soup to taste.

Nutritional values:

Calories/Energy: 61 Kcal, Protein: 3.2 g (19.4%), Carbs: 9.88 g (64.7%), Lipids: 1.09 g (15.9%), Fibbers: 1.9 g, Calcium: 12 mg, Phosphorous: 47 mg, Potassium: 71 mg, Sodium: 336 mg

83. Tomato soup made from fresh tomatoes

Ingredients (for 2 people):

- 1 kg of tomatoes
- 200 ml of water
- ½ teaspoon salt
- 1 sprig of rosemary
- 1 sprig of thyme
- 2 tbsp cream
- 2 tbsp sour cream

Preparation:

1. Wash the tomatoes and put them in a saucepan with water and salt. Bring to a boil. Simmer for 10-15 minutes, until the peel starts to peel off the tomatoes and the tomatoes are soft.
2. In the meantime, wash the herbs and let them dry on kitchen paper.
3. Drain the tomatoes, collecting the cooking water if necessary. Strain or strain the soft tomatoes through a sieve. Let the pureed tomatoes simmer for about 10 minutes. Then stir with the cream until smooth. Dilute with some of the collected cooking water as desired.
4. Strip off the rosemary and thyme needles and chop finely. Pour the soup into two bowls, put a dollop of sour cream on top and sprinkle everything with the herbs.

Nutritional values:

186 kcal, 6 g protein, 8 g fat, 21 g carbohydrates, 2 g fibbers

84. Chickpea soup with croutons

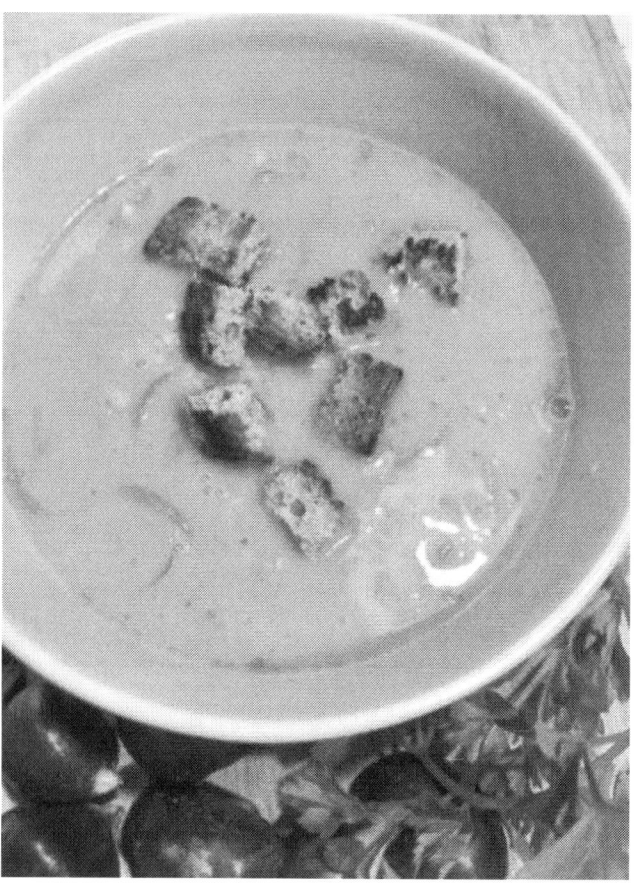

Serving: 1 – 4

Ingredients:

- (FOR EACH PERSON)
- Dried chickpeas 60 g
- Common bread without salt 80 g
- Extra virgin olive oil 20 g
- Rosemary
- Sage
- Garlic
- Bay leaf
- Chilli

Preparation:

1. Soak the chickpeas the night before.
2. Put two pots of water on the stove and bring to a boil.

3. Meanwhile, prepare a sauté with chopped rosemary, a bit of garlic, oil, sage, a few bay leaves, and a little chili. When the garlic is golden, it should be removed.
4. Pour the chickpeas into boiling water, drain them after a quarter of an hour and dip them back into the second pot of boiling water. Leave to cook for another quarter of an hour.
5. Add some chickpeas to the mixture and place them in a small pan with some of their water. The others must be blended to create a cream that we can make more or less thick with the addition of your water. Add the whole chickpeas, bring to the boil again and add the common pasta.
6. Serve accompanied with common wood baked toasted bread, adding a drizzle of extra virgin olive oil.

Nutritional values:

Water: 150 g, Protein: 23 g, Phosphorous: 241mg, Potassium: 609 mg, lipids: 23 g, Carbs: 81 g, Sodium: 8 mg, Calories: 594 kcal

85. Chestnut and chickpea soup

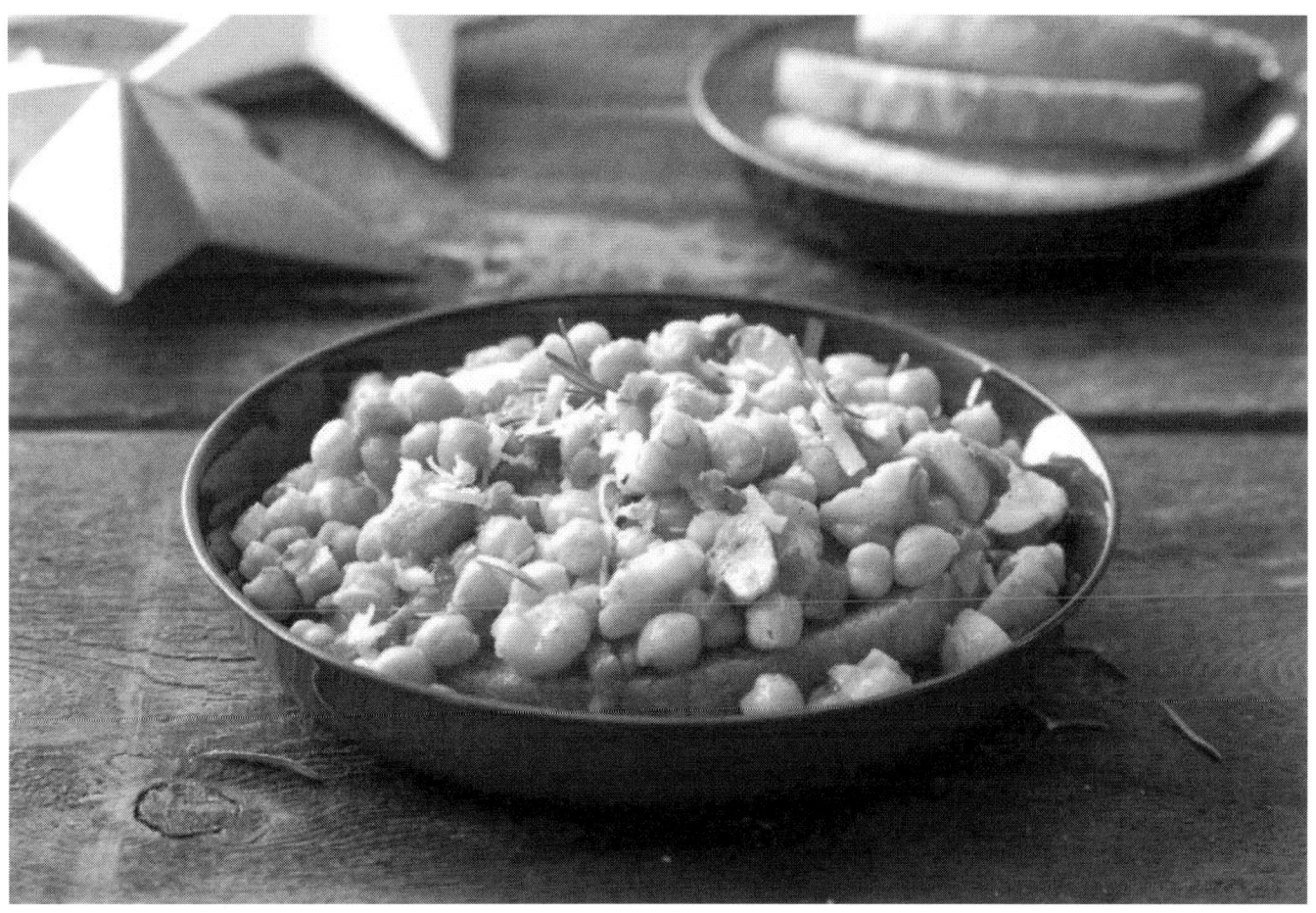

Serving: 6

Ingredients:

- Dried chickpeas 300 g
- Chestnuts without peel 250 g
- Extra virgin olive oil 40 g
- A hint of tomato paste
- 2 cloves of garlic
- Rosemary
- Water 1500 cc
- Fresh pasta 100 g

Preparation:

1. To prepare this recipe, calculate that you need to soak the chickpeas for a whole night. The next morning, drain the chickpeas, transfer them to a saucepan and cover with cold water. After a first boil, replace the water with just as boiling, resume cooking, and let them cook over low heat for about 2 hours, until tender.
2. Meanwhile, boil the chestnuts too. Then peel them and mash some.
3. In a large pot, put the chopped garlic and rosemary needles; fry in 2 tablespoons of oil for a few minutes then add the whole chestnuts and the crushed ones. Add the tomato puree, water, and, after a few minutes, the chickpeas. Let it boil for about another hour. Add the squares and cook. Serve with a drizzle of raw extra virgin olive oil.
4. You can serve the soup with slices of toasted bread instead of pasta.

The original recipe calls for chestnuts to be cooked in the oven. To speed up the preparation, I used already peeled and frozen chestnuts. You can also use canned boiled chickpeas. Drain them from the preserving liquid to eliminate part of the potassium. In this case, the sodium increases, as canned chickpeas contain salt. The reported potassium value is calculated with raw chickpeas and chestnuts. When cooking in water, the actual value is reduced. Beware if you have problems with potassium. In conservative therapy and transplantation, it can be a tasty single dish.

Nutritional values:

Water: 279 g, Protein: 14 g, Phosphorous: 215 mg, Potassium: 635 mg, Lipids: 10 g, Carbs: 56 g, Sodium: 17 mg, Calories: 359 kcal

CHAPTER TEN: Salads

86. Hawaiian Chicken Salad

Number of serving 4, total cooking time 30mins

Ingredients:

- 1 1/2 cups of chicken breast, cooked, chopped
- 1 cup pineapple chunks, canned, drained
- 1 1/4 cups lettuce iceberg, shredded
- 1/2 cup celery, diced
- 1/2 cup mayonnaise
- 1/8 tsp (dash) Tabasco sauce
- 2 lemon juice
- 1/4 tsp black pepper

Preparation:

1. Combine the cooked chicken, pineapple, lettuce, and celery in a medium bowl. Just set aside.
2. In a small bowl, make the dressing. Mix the mayonnaise, Tabasco sauce, pepper, and lemon juice.
3. Use the chicken mixture to add the dressing and stir until well mixed.

Nutrient Analysis:

Power: 310 g, Protein: 16.8 g, Carbohydrates: 9.6 g, fibbers: 1.1 g, Fat: 23.1 g, Sodium: 200 mg, Potassium: 260 mg, Phosphorus: 134 mg

87. Grated carrot salad with lemon-Dijon vinaigrette

Servings: 8; Preparation: 15 min

Ingredients:

- 9 small carrots (14 cm), peeled
- 2 tbsp. 1/2 teaspoon Dijon mustard
- 1 C. lemon juice
- 2 tbsp. extra virgin olive oil
- 1-2 tsp. honey (to taste)
- ¼ tsp. salt
- ¼ tsp. freshly ground pepper (to taste)
- 2 tbsp. chopped parsley

- 1 green onion, thinly sliced

Preparation:

1. Grate the carrots in a food processor. Book.
2. In a salad bowl, mix Dijon mustard, lemon juice, honey, olive oil, salt, and pepper. Add the carrots, fresh parsley, and green onions. Stir to coat well. Cover and refrigerate until ready to serve.

If your carrots are more or less sweet, adjust the touch of honey.

Nutrient Analysis:

Energy: 61 g, Proteins: 1 g, Carbohydrates: 7 g, fibbers: 1 g, Total Fat: 4 g, Sodium: 88 mg, Phosphorus: 22 mg, Potassium: 197 mg

88. Tuna macaroni salad

Ingredients:

- 1 1/2 cups Uncooked Macaroni
- 1 170g Can of tuna in water
- 1/4 cup Mayonnaise
- 2 medium celery stalks, diced
- 1 Tbsp. Lemon Pepper Seasoning

Preparation:

1. Cook the pasta and let it cool in the refrigerator.
2. Drain the tuna in a colander and rinse it with cold water.
3. Add the tuna and celery once the macaroni has cooled.
4. Stir in mayonnaise and sprinkle with lemon seasoning. Mix well. Serve cold.

Nutrient Analysis:

Power: 136 g, Protein: 8.0 g, Carbohydrates: 18 g, fibbers: 0.8 g, Fat: 3.6 g, Sodium: 75 mg, Potassium: 124 mg, Phosphorus: 90 mg

89. Couscous salad

Ingredients:

- 3 cups of water
- 1/2 tsp. cinnamon tea
- 1/2 tsp. cumin tea
- 1 tsp. honey soup

- 2 tbsp. lemon juice
- 3 cups quick-cooking couscous
- 2 tbsp. tea of olive oil
- 1 green onion,
- Finely chopped 1 small carrot, finely diced
- 1/2 red pepper,
- Finely diced fresh coriander

Preparation:

1. Stir in the water with the cinnamon, cumin, honey, and lemon juice and bring to a boil. Put the couscous in it, cover it, and remove it from the heat. To swell the couscous, stir with a fork. Add the vegetables, fresh herbs, and olive oil. It is possible to serve the salad warm or cold.

Nutrient Analysis:

Energy: 190 g, Protein: 6 g, Carbohydrates: 38 g, fibbers: 2 g, Total Fat: 1 g, Sodium: 4 mg, Phosphorus: 82 mg, Potassium: 116 mg

90. Fruity zucchini salad

Servings: 4

Ingredients:

- 400g zucchini
- 1 small onion
- 4 tbsp olive oil
- 100g pineapple preserve, drained
- Salt, paprika
- thyme

Preparation:

Dice the onions and sauté in the oil until translucent. Cut the zucchini into slices and add. Season with salt, paprika, and thyme. Let cool and mix with the cut pineapple.

Nutritional values per serving:

Energy: 150kcal, Protein: 2g, Fat: 10g, Carbohydrates: 10g, Dietary fibbers: 2g, Potassium: 220mg, Calcium: 38mg, Phosphate: 24mg

91. Cucumber salad, pulled through slowly

Servings 4

Ingredients:

- 1 cucumber
- 1 tbsp salt
- 100 ml of water
- 100 ml white wine vinegar
- 2 tbsp cane sugar
- 5 peppercorns, crushed
- 1/2 teaspoon cinnamon
- 1/2 teaspoon of allspice
- 1 teaspoon chili powder
- 1 teaspoon ginger powder

Preparation:

The salad has to brew a day before it is eaten, so start early! Wash the cucumber and cut it into thin slices, put them in a bowl, sprinkle with salt and stir, shake well so that the salt gets everywhere. Then let it steep for half an hour. Meanwhile, in a saucepan, mix water, vinegar, sugar, pepper, cinnamon, allspice, chili, and ginger and bring to the boil once, then let cool again with the lid closed. Rinse the lettuce slices and pour off the water. If necessary, dry in a towel. Add the dressing from the pot to the salad slices and let everything sit in the fridge for a day.

Nutritional values per serving:

Energy: 49kcal, Protein: 1g, Carbohydrates: 5g, Potassium: 234mg, Sodium: 500mg, Calcium: 34mg, Phosphate: 21mg

92. Tortellini salad

Servings: 4

Ingredients:

- 200g tortellini with meat filling
- 100g red peppers
- 1 tomato
- 1 clove of garlic
- Salt pepper
- fresh basil, some leaves

- 3 tbsp rapeseed oil
- 1 tbsp white wine vinegar

Preparation:

1. Cook the tortellini in salted water according to the instructions on the packet and drain.
2. Finely dice the peppers and garlic and sweat in the rapeseed oil. Add the vinegar and spices and pour over the tortellini. Cut the tomato into small pieces and mix in. Mix with the fresh basil and season to taste.

Nutritional values per serving:

Energy: 161kcal, Protein: 4g, Fat: 9g, Carbohydrates: 18g, Dietary fibbers: 3g, Potassium: 173mg, Phosphate: 80mg

93. Farmer's Salad

Servings: 2

Ingredients:

- 60g mixed leaf salads
- 100g red pepper, diced
- 200g green beans, canned, drained
- 60g feta cheese
- 1 tbsp wine vinegar
- 1 tbsp diced onions
- Salt, pepper, sugar
- 2 tbsp olive oil

Preparation:

1. Mix vinegar with onions, oil, and spices and mix with the salad. Cut the sheep's cheese into cubes and serve with the salad.
2. It goes well with baguette or flatbread with herb butter.

Nutritional values per serving:

Energy: 187kcal, Protein: 8g, Fat: 16g, Carbohydrates: 4g, Dietary fibbers: 5g, Potassium: 396mg, Calcium: 188mg, Phosphate: 170mg

94. Orange and grapefruit salad with date stripes

Preparation time 20mins, total time 40mins, serving 2

Ingredients:

- 125 g small organic orange (1 small organic orange)
- 175 g small pink grapefruit (organic quality, 1 small pink grapefruit)
- 1 dried date

Preparation steps:

1. Rinse orange and grapefruit with hot water and rub dry.
2. Use a peeler to peel off an approx. 3 cm long strip of peel from both fruits very thinly and cut across into fine strips.
3. Peel the orange and grapefruit thick enough to remove the white skin.
4. Cut out the fruit fillets between the separating skins; work over a bowl and catch the juice.
5. Halve the date lengthways, remove the stone if necessary, cut the pulp into very fine strips.
6. Mix the date strips with the fruit fillets, half of the peel strips, and the captured juice in a bowl. Let it steep for 10 minutes. Arrange on a plate and sprinkle with the remaining strips of peel.

Nutritional values:

Calories 100 kcal (5%), Protein 2 g (2%), Fat 0 g (0%), Carbohydrates 20 g (13%), added sugar 0 g (0%), fibbers 3 g (10%)

95. Chicken and asparagus salad with watercress

Preparation 40mins serving 4

Ingredients:

- 100 g spring onions (0.5 bunch)
- 200 g cherry tomatoes
- 100 g green asparagus
- 600 g chicken breast fillet (4 chicken breast fillets)
- salt
- pepper
- 1 small lime
- 1 clove of garlic
- 6 tbsp honey
- 1 tbsp grainy mustard
- 5 tbsp olive oil

- 100 g watercress

Preparation steps:

1. The spring onions are cleaned and washed and then cut into thin rings. Wash the tomatoes and quarter them.
2. The woody ends of the asparagus are cut off. Wash and pat the asparagus to dry. Halve the sticks and, with a peeler, cut the halves lengthwise into thin slices.
3. Wash the fillets of chicken, pat them dry with kitchen paper, and cut them into strips. With salt and pepper, season.
4. Trim the lime in half for the dressing and squeeze out the juice. Peel the garlic and dice it. Mix the mustard, 3 tablespoons of lime juice, and 3 tablespoons of oil with the honey. With salt and pepper, season.
5. In a large non-stick pan, heat the remaining oil and stir-fry the meat over high heat for about 5 minutes.
6. In a bowl, add the chicken, spring onions, tomatoes, and asparagus. Mix in the dressing and allow the salad to steep for 10 minutes or so.
7. Meanwhile, wash the cress and shake it dry. Pluck the leaves, chop coarsely as desired, and spread on dishes or bowls. Use salt and pepper to season the chicken salad and serve on the cress.

Nutritional values:

Calories 368 kcal (18%), Protein 37 g (38%), Fat 14 g (12%), Carbohydrates 22 g (15%), added sugar 17 g (68%), fibbers 2 g (7%)

96. Buckwheat salad

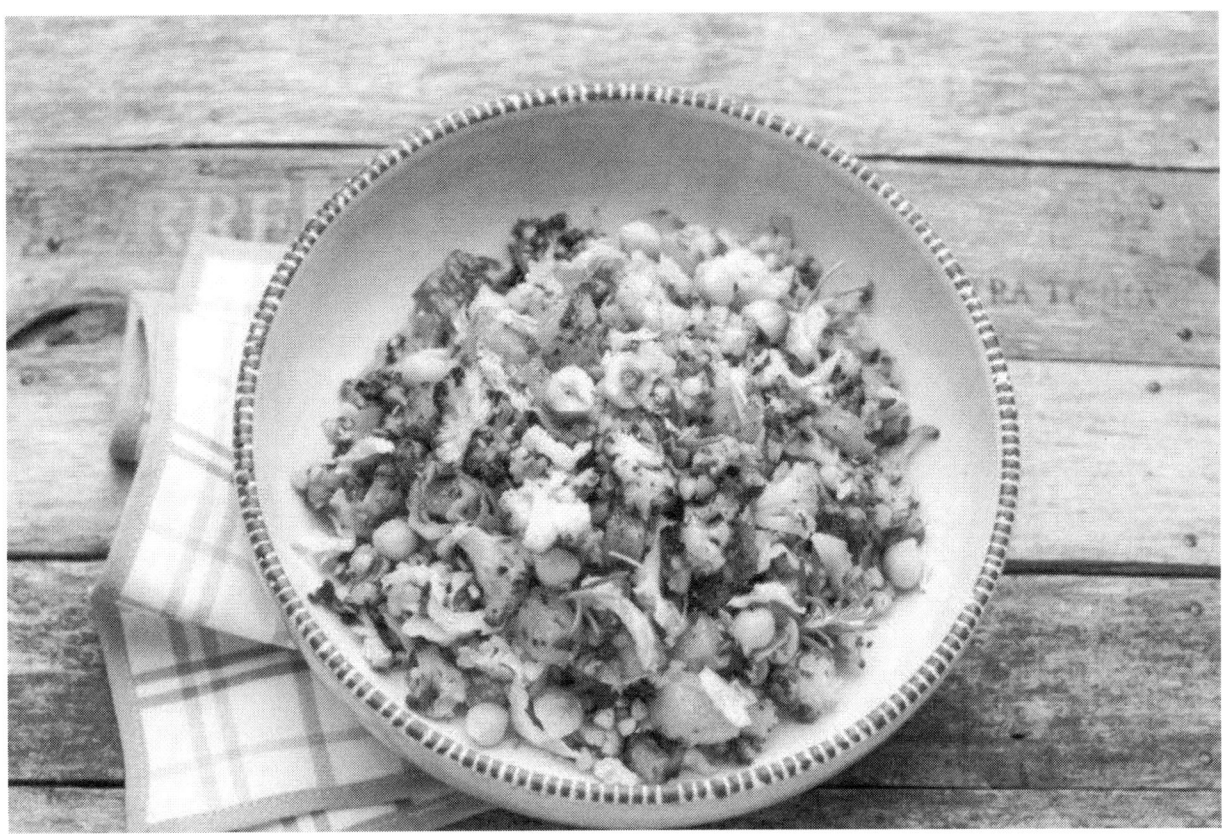

Serving: 4

Ingredients:

- Buckwheat 300 g
- Carrots 300 g
- Cherry tomatoes 250 g
- Feta cheese 200 g
- Pitted green olives 80 g
- Extra virgin olive oil 60 g
- Pickled capers 20 g
- Fresh chives
- Fresh mint

Preparation:

1. I boiled the buckwheat in plenty of water for 20 minutes.
2. In the meantime, I have steamed the previously peeled carrots.
3. In a bowl I collected the feta cut into cubes, the tomatoes cut into small wedges; the chopped capers. I added the diced carrots and the cooled buckwheat.

4. I seasoned with plenty of extra virgin olive oil, chopped chives, and mint and I turned well. I let it cook for about 2 hours.

Buckwheat is rich in complex carbohydrates and fibbers. For this reason, blood sugar rises more slowly and is suitable for those with diabetes. It is also gluten-free and can also be used by those suffering from celiac disease. In this recipe, the high sodium is related to feta. If you leave it to flavour, thanks also to the herbs, you don't need to add more!

Nutritional values:

Water: 300 g, Protein: 19 g, Phosphorous: 448 mg, Potassium: 847 mg, Lipids: 31 g, Carbs: 63 g, Sodium: 883 mg, Calories: 585 kcal

97. Salad with feta and taggiasca olives

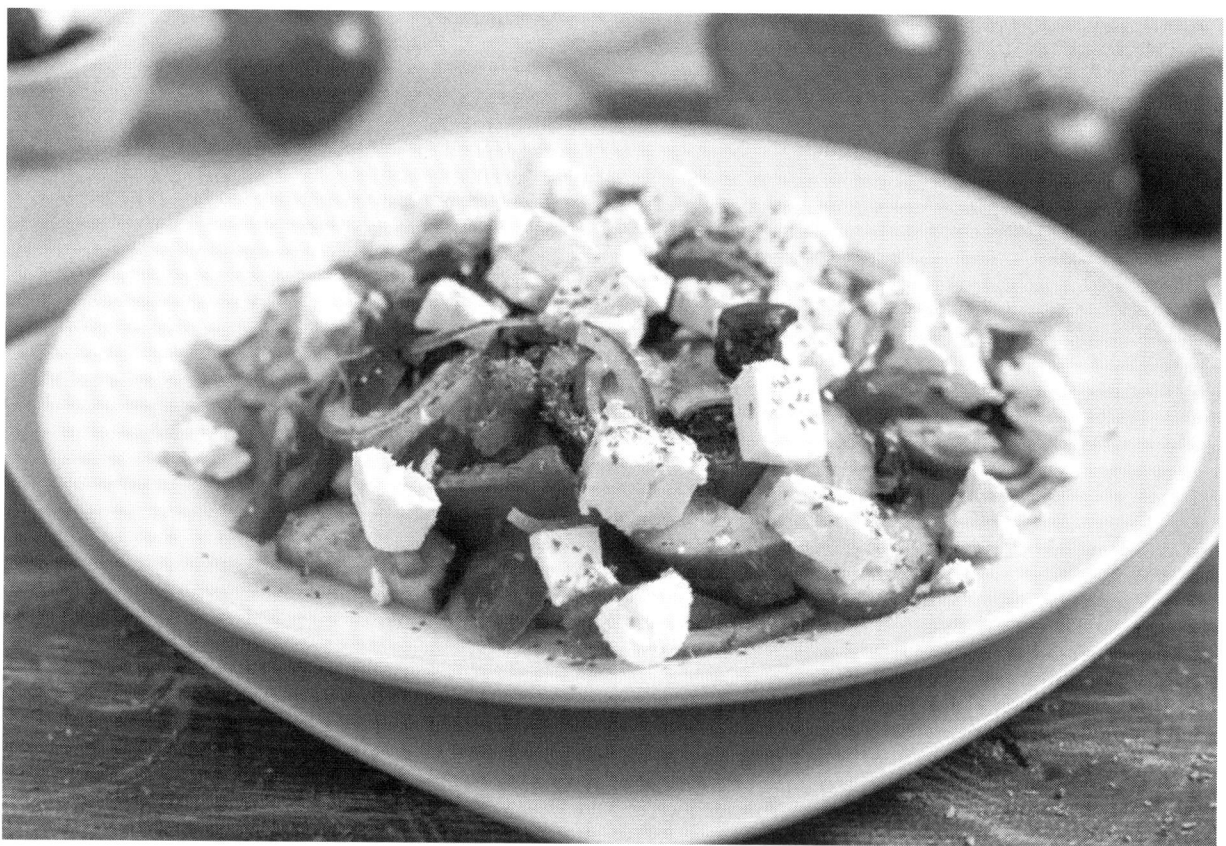

Serving: 1 - 4

Ingredients:

- Salad tomatoes 100 g
- Cucumbers 100 g
- Feta cheese 100 g
- 10 g taggiasca olives

- Extra virgin olive oil 10 g
- Onion if you like
- Oregano and fresh basil
- Common bread without salt 100 g

Preparation:

1. Wash the vegetables, peel the cucumber, and cut everything into small pieces.
2. Season with oregano, chopped basil, and olives. If you like, add finely chopped onion.
3. Add the feta cheese cut into chunks, drizzle with oil, and mix.
4. Eat accompanying with unsalted bread.

There is no need to add salt because the feta and olives already bring too much. Consuming with bread without salt allows you not to add further and completes the dish. This salad is also high in phosphorus - nearly half the desirable daily amount. So, remember to take the chelators!

Nutritional values:

Water: 282 g, Protein: 27 g, Phosphorous: 401 mg, Potassium: 687 mg, Lipids: 34 g, Carbs: 67 g, Sodium: 1582 mg, Calories: 662 kcal

98. Kartoffelsalat

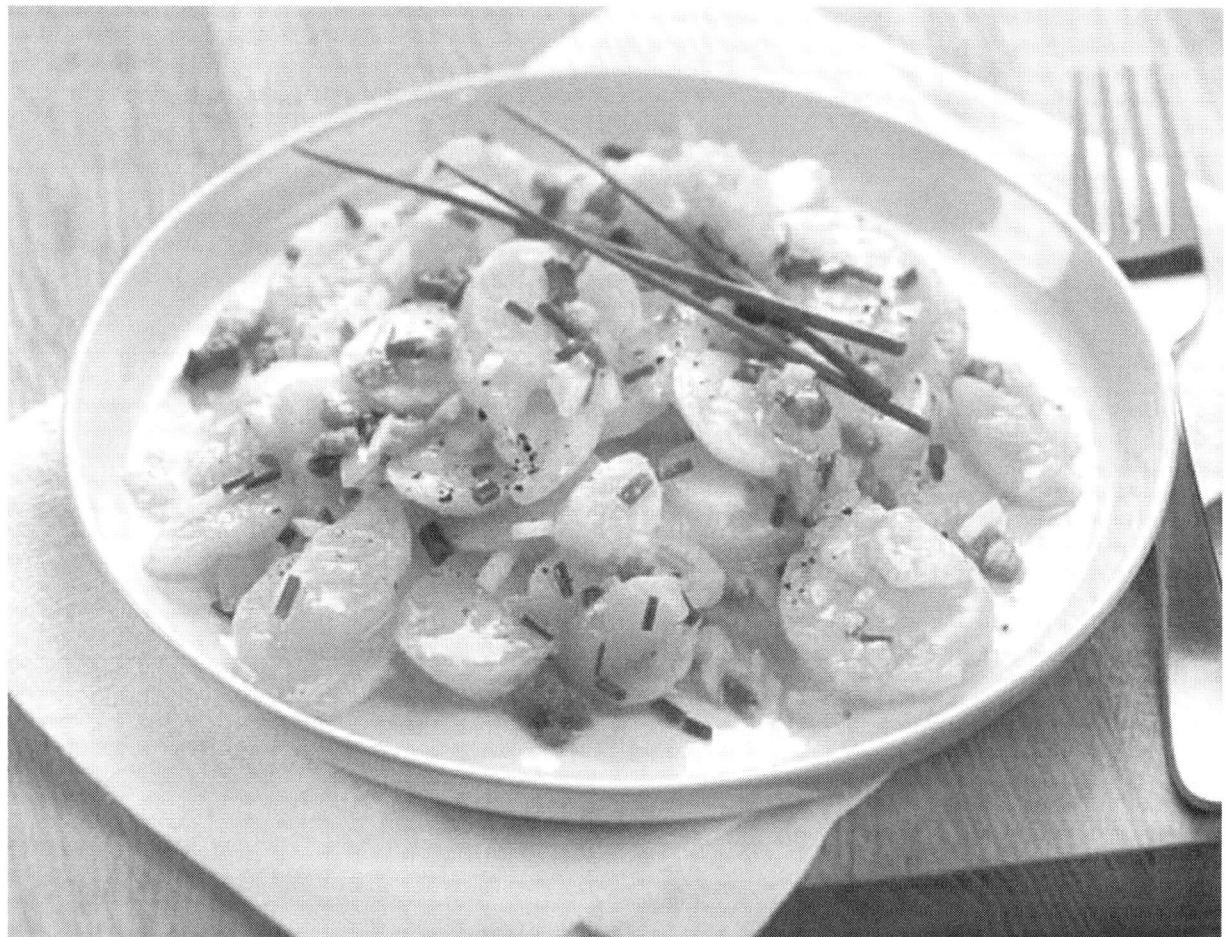

Serving: 6

Ingredients:

- Potatoes 1200 g
- Sweet and sour cucumbers 150 g
- 2 eggs
- Red apple 150 g
- Sausage 100 g
- Extra virgin olive oil 80 g
- (FOR THE BRINE)
- Onion 150 g
- 125 cc of vinegar
- 125 cc of water
- Sugar 15 g
- Salt and pepper

Preparation:

4. Boil the potatoes, drain and peel them. When they are cold, cut them into pieces.
5. Prepare the brine. Finely chop the onion. Put it in a saucepan and cover with vinegar and water, sugar, salt, and pepper and boil for 5 minutes. You will have to pour it hot over the potatoes.
6. Boil the eggs and cut them into wedges. Cut the sausages into small pieces. Cut the cucumbers into slices. Wash the red apple well and cut it into slices without peeling.
7. In a dish, combine all the ingredients and season with extra virgin olive oil. Mix gently.
8. Cover the plate with cling film and leave to flavour for a few hours in the refrigerator.

A gorgeous potato salad! To be prepared in advance. A single dish for conservative and transplantation. Rich in potassium. If you have trouble, peel the potatoes, cut them into small pieces, soak them in plenty of water overnight, and then boil them in plenty of water - but leave the potatoes a little tough. Or make up for the day.

Nutritional values:

Water: 262 g, Protein: 10 g, Phosphorous: 193 mg, Potassium: 1294 mg, Lipids: 21 g, Carbs: 43 g, Sodium: 352 mg, Calories: 392 kcal

CHAPTER ELEVEN: Vegetarian Recipes

99. Spring vegetables with tofu from the wok

Ingredients for 4 persons:

- 500 g green asparagus
- alternatively: 2 yellow or red peppers
- 1 bunch of spring onions
- 350 g pointed cabbage
- 1 bowl of watercress
- 1 package (100 g) mixed sprouts
- 25 g fresh ginger
- 2 cloves of garlic
- 1 dried chili pepper
- 3-4 tbsp soy sauce
- 3 tbsp lime juice
- 4 tbsp oil
- 300 g tofu
- to turn: wholemeal spelled flour

Preparation:

1. Wash the asparagus, cut off the woody ends, slice the stalks into pieces about 2 cm wide. Wash, core, and, alternatively, cut the peppers into suitable pieces.
2. Clean, wash, and cut the spring onions into pieces. It cleans and washes pointed cabbage, cutting out the stalk. Cut fine cabbage strips. Clean, dry, spin, and wash. Plug them into bits bite-sized. Peel and chop ginger and garlic. Dried chili crumbles. Combine in a bowl, soy sauce, and lime juice. Add the sesame oil.
3. Heat a wok or deep pan with 2 tablespoons of oil. Cut the tofu into bite-sized pieces and mix with some wholemeal flour. Fry in hot oil until brown. Season with salt and pepper. Use kitchen paper to remove/drain. Drain that oil.
4. Heat the remaining wok oil. Fry asparagus for 1-2 minutes while stirring. Fry onions and cabbage and the remaining vegetables for a minute. Combine marinade, fold pieces of tofu. Season with salt and pepper.

Nutritional values per serving:

383 kcal, 24 g fat, 20 g carbohydrates, 22 g protein, 8 g fibbers, 1.7

100. Asparagus and carrot salad with burrata

Preparation time 15mins, total time 30mins, serving 2

Ingredients:

- 250 g white asparagus
- 250 g green asparagus
- 2 carrots
- 3 tbsp olive oil
- 1 tbsp sunflower seeds
- 1 tbsp lemon juice
- 150 g cherry tomatoes
- 1 handful arugula
- 1 spring onion
- 2 bullets burrata

Preparation steps:

1. Peel the asparagus and the lower ends are cut off. Wash the green asparagus and the woody ends are also cut off. Cut it into pieces with the asparagus. Clean, peel, and cut into sticks with the carrots.
2. In a saucepan, heat the oil and fry the asparagus and carrots over medium heat for five minutes. Add the seeds to the sunflower and roast for 3 minutes. Deglaze with lemon juice and add salt and pepper to season the asparagus and carrot mix. Take it off the stove then and let it cool down.
3. Wash the tomatoes and quarter them at the same time. Rocket wash and dry shake. The spring onions are cleaned, washed, and cut into pieces.
4. Mix the tomatoes, rocket, and spring onions with the asparagus, arrange them on plates and serve each with a scoop of burrata.

Nutritional values:

Calories 671 kcal (32%), Protein 34 g (35%), Fat 48 g (41%), Carbohydrates 26 g (17%), added sugar 0 g (0%), fibbers 9.4 g (31%)

101. Quinoa Salad Winning

Cooking time 1h, serving 4

Ingredients:

- 200 g quinoa

- 1 mango
- 1 cucumber
- 3 tomatoes
- 1 red pepper
- 150 g lamb's lettuce
- 1 red onion
- 2 stems mint
- 150 g feta (45% fat in dry matter)
- 1 tbsp olive oil
- 1 tbsp apple cider vinegar
- salt
- pepper

Preparation steps:

1. Rinse the quinoa with cold water, bring to the boil in a saucepan with twice the amount of water and cook over low heat for about 10 minutes. In the meantime, peel the mango, cut from the stone, and dice the pulp. Clean, wash and cut the cucumber, tomatoes, and peppers. Wash the lamb's lettuce and spin dry. Peel and chop the onion. Wash the mint, shake dry, pluck the leaves and cut into strips. Dice the feta.
2. Drain the quinoa, drain and transfer to a bowl. Add the mango, cucumber, tomatoes, bell pepper, lamb's lettuce, onion, mint, and feta and mix. Season the salad with olive oil, apple cider vinegar, salt, and pepper.

Nutritional values:

Calories 409 kcal (19%), Protein 15 g (15%), Fat 16 g (14%), Carbohydrates 50 g (33%), added sugar 0 g (0%), fibbers 8.9 g (30%)

102. Spinach Mango Vegetables

Preparation time 40mins, serving 2

Ingredients:

- 750 g young spinach leaves
- 200 g spring onions (2 bunch)
- 800 g ripe mango (2 ripe mangoes)
- 2 tbsp germ oil
- 30 g ginger (1 piece)
- 30 g sunflower seeds (2 tbsp)
- 20 g amaranth pops

- salt
- cayenne pepper

Preparation steps:

1. Thoroughly wash the spinach, spin it dry and clean.
2. The spring onions are cleaned and washed and cut into pieces about 2 cm wide.
3. The mangoes peel. Slice the stone pulp and cut it into cubes about 1 cm in size.
4. In a saucepan, heat 1 tablespoon of oil and cook the covered spring onions over medium heat for about 5 minutes. Add the spinach and cook for about 5 minutes, covered.
5. Meanwhile, peel the ginger and finely grate it, collecting the juice.
6. Add the spinach to the mango cubes, ginger and ginger juice, and cover and heat for about 3 minutes over medium heat.
7. Meanwhile, in a coated pan, heat the remaining oil. Roast the seeds of the sunflower for 3-4 minutes over low heat, add the pops of amaranth, and heat briefly.
8. Season the salted spinach and mango vegetables and arrange them on a plate. Sprinkle over the vegetables and season the roasted sunflower seeds and amaranth pops with cayenne pepper.

Nutritional values:

Calories 240 kcal (11%), Protein 8 g (8%), Fat 10 g (9%), Carbohydrates 27 g (18%), added sugar 0 g (0%), fibbers 9.5 g (32%)

103. Braised Swiss chard with garlic and balsamic vinegar

Total time 30mins, preparation time 15mins, serving 2

Ingredients:

- 1 large bunch of Swiss chard
- 1 tbsp. to s. olive oil
- 2 cloves of garlic, minced
- 1/4 tsp. red pepper flakes
- 1 tbsp balsamic vinegar or lemon juice

Preparation:

1. Clean the leaves and cut their base.
2. Add oil and garlic to a preheated skillet. Add the chilies and leaves, then stir over high heat until the leaves are tender. Add vinegar or lemon juice. Serve with crushed pepper.

Nutrient Analysis:

Energy: 88 g, Protein: 1.4 g, Carbohydrates: 5.4 g, Total Fat: 7 g, Sodium: 165 mg, Phosphorus: 42 mg, Potassium: 314 mg

104. Snow peas all with thyme

Servings: 4

Ingredients:

- 2 tbsp. at t. (10 mL) margarine
- 2 tbsp. at t. (10 mL) fresh lemon juice
- Zest of one lemon
- 1 tsp. at t. (5 mL) dried thyme
- ½ pound (250 g) snow peas, trimmed

Preparation:

1. Melt the margarine in a shallow pot.
2. Combine lemon zest and juice, and thyme set aside.
3. Steam the snow peas for 3 minutes over boiling water or in the microwave on high for 3 minutes until tender.
4. Drain and fold into the mixture.

Nutrient Analysis:

Energy: 45 g, Proteins: 2 g, Carbohydrates: 5 g, fibbers: 1.7 g, Total Fat: 2.4 g, Sodium: 30 mg, Phosphorus: 42.6 mg, Potassium: 296 mg

105. Cauliflower and fresh dill

Serving 2, preparation time 30mins

Ingredients:

- 1 medium cauliflower head
- 2 tbsp. to s. (25 mL) lemon juice
- 1 tbsp. to s. (15 mL) olive oil
- 1/3 cup (75 mL) fresh dill, chopped
- Pepper to taste

Preparation:

1. The leaves and stems are removed from the cauliflower; the florets are cut.

2. Cook in a large pot of boiling water, cover for 10 minutes or until tender; drain out the cauliflower.
3. Transfer to a dish for serving.
4. Mix the oil with the lemon juice; pour the cauliflower over it and mix.
5. Sprinkle with dill and sprinkle with pepper to taste.

Nutrient Analysis:

Energy: 45 g, Proteins: 2 g, Carbohydrates: 5 g, fibbers: 1.7 g, Total Fat: 2.4 g, Sodium: 30 mg, Phosphorus: 42.6 mg, Potassium: 296 mg

106. Zucchini and corn stir-fry

Ingredients:

- 2 medium zucchinis, diced
- 2 cups frozen corn
- 1 medium red pepper, diced
- 1 Tbsp. at t. chili flakes
- 1 tbsp. to s. vegetable oil

Preparation:

1. Heat the oil in a pan.
2. Add vegetables and chili, cook over high heat until zucchini is tender.

Nutrient Analysis:

Energy: 67 g, Proteins: 2 g, Carbohydrates: 11 g, fibbers: 1.6 g, Total Fat: 2 g, Sodium: 6 mg, Phosphorus: 53 mg, Potassium: 253 mg

107. Marinated zucchini

Serving: 1 - 8

Ingredients:

- Zucchini 500 g
- Extra virgin olive oil 30 g
- 4 tablespoons of lemon juice
- 4 tablespoons of apple (or rice) cider vinegar
- 2 cloves of garlic
- 2 sprigs of mint
- 1 dry chili
- 1 pinch of salt

Preparation:

1. Wash the courgettes well, check the two ends, and cut them into very thin slices lengthwise using a mandolin or a potato peeler.
2. Wash the mint and dry it, remove a few leaves that you will keep whole, and chop the rest of the leaves.
3. For the marinade, mix the lemon with the vinegar and oil in a bowl, add the chopped mint, salt, and crumbled red pepper.
4. In a rectangular container, of suitable length, arrange the courgette slices lined up in layers and season with the marinade, alternating between the layers a few pieces of garlic and a few whole mint leaves.
5. Close the container and let it rest in the refrigerator for at least 5 hours. Remove from the refrigerator 10 minutes before serving.
6. In a tightly closed glass container, they can be kept in the refrigerator for up to a couple of days.

A fresh summer appetizer. Zucchini must be very fresh, possibly small, and without seeds.

Nutritional values:

Protein: 2 g, Calories: 81 kcal, Potassium 5 *, Low Phosphorus, Lipids: 7 g, Cholesterol: 0 mg

108. "Cooked water"

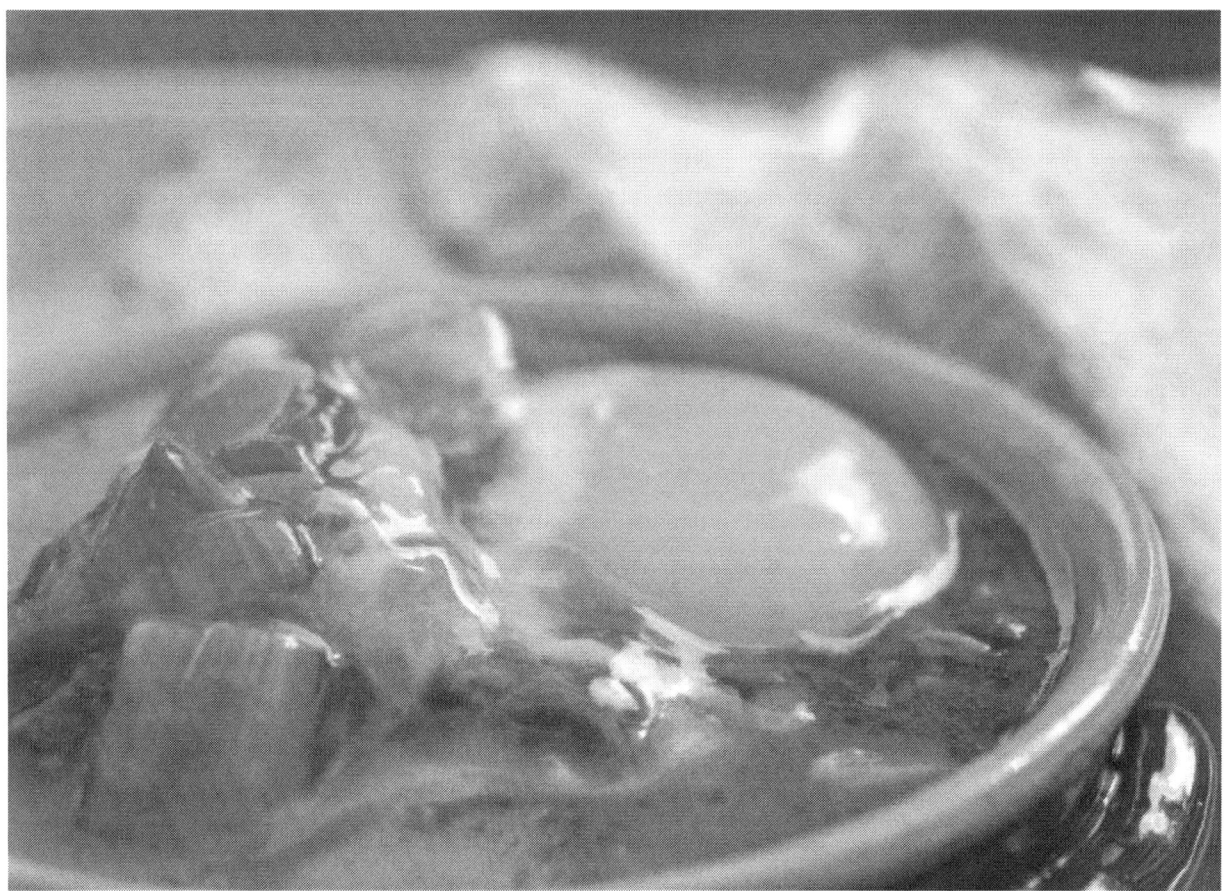

Serving: 4

Ingredients:

- Potatoes 400 g
- Field chicory 300 g
- Artichokes n 4 (about 200 g clean)
- Onion 100 g
- Ripe tomatoes 100 g
- Onion 100 g
- Garlic 3-4 cloves
- Chilli
- Mint
- 4 eggs
- Unsalted bread 200 g
- Extra virgin olive oil 40 g

Preparation:

1. Put the peeled and halved potatoes, the cleaned and halved artichokes, 3-4 whole garlic cloves, the sliced onions, the mint, the chili pepper, and the chopped tomatoes in a saucepan with only water and salt. Cook for about 1 hour.
2. If you use wild chicory, you will have to blanch it separately for a few minutes to eliminate the bitter and not everyone's taste. Add it later to the preparation. If you use the cultivated one, you can add it from the beginning.
3. When cooked, add one egg per person, poached in the broth of the same soup.
4. During cooking, you have to pay attention to keep a certain amount of liquid by adding hot water. When cooked, pour the broth on the bread making sure you have all the ingredients for each dish.
5. Let it rest for a few minutes with the plate covered, so that the bread can get wet properly, then throw away the liquid not absorbed by the bread and sprinkle the soup abundantly with extra virgin olive oil.

Cooked in water without sautéing and without the presence of animal fats because it is dedicated to vegetarian customers, it is representative of the Mediterranean diet. In conservative therapy or transplantation, it can be considered as a complete "single dish" thanks to the addition of the egg. For those who have problems with potassium: be careful because it is very rich in it!

Nutritional values:

Water: 557 g, Protein: 17 g, Phosphorous: 306 mg, Potassium: 1296 mg, Lipids: 17 g, Carbs: 54 g, Sodium: 209 mg, Calories: 429 kcal

CHAPTER TWELVE: Desserts and Sweets

109. Oatmeal and berry muffins

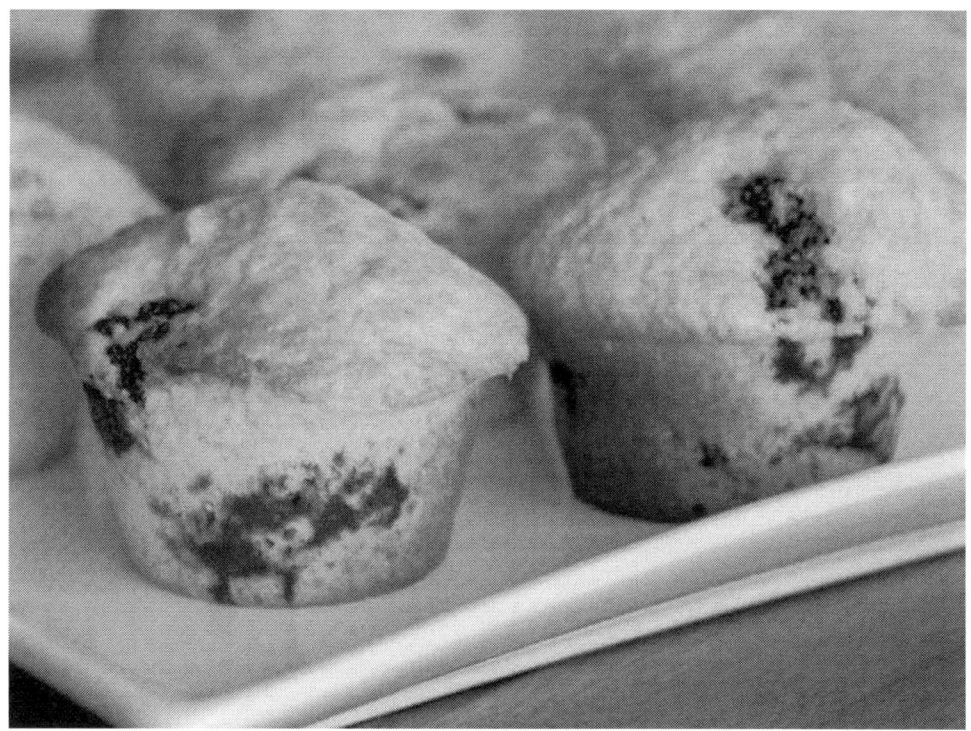

Cooking time 40mins, total time 60mins, serving 6

Ingredients:

- 1 cup (250 mL) non-blanched all-purpose flour
- ½ cup (125 mL) quick-cooking oatmeal 1/2 cup
- (160 mL) stuffed brown sugar
- 1/2 tbsp (1/2 cup) tea) baking soda
- 2 eggs
- 125 ml (1/2 cup) applesauce
- 60 ml (1/4 cup)
- Orange canola oil 1, grated rind only
- 1 lemon, grated rind
- 15 ml (1 tbsp) lemon juice
- 180 ml (3/4 cup) fresh raspberries (see note)
- 180 ml (3/4 cup) fresh or blueberries (or blackberries)

Preparation:

1. Put the grill at the centre of the oven. Preheat oven to 180 ° C (350 ° F). Line 12 muffin cups with paper or silicone trays.
2. In a bowl, combine flour, oatmeal, brown sugar, and baking soda. Book.
3. In a big bowl, whisk together eggs, applesauce, oil, citrus zest, and lemon juice. Add the dry ingredients to the wooden spoon. Add the berries and mix gently.
4. Spread the mixture in the boxes. Sprinkle top with pistachio muffins. Bake for 20 to 22 minutes or until a toothpick inserted in the centre of a muffin comes out clean. Let cool.

Nutritional values:

Calories: 320.54 kcal, Carbohydrates: 45.18 g, Protein: 7.06 g, Fat: 13.69 g, Sodium: 359.94 mg, fibbers: 3.08 g

110. Crunchy Blueberry and Apples

Cooking time 10mins, total time 50mins, serving 4

Ingredients:

Crunchy

- 1 cup (1¼ cup) quick-cooking oatmeal
- ¼ cup (60 mL) brown sugar
- ¼ cup (60 mL) unbleached all-purpose flour
- 90 ml (6 tablespoons) melted margarine

Garnish

- 125 ml (½ cup) brown sugar
- 20 ml (4 teaspoons) corn starch
- 1 litter (4 cups) fresh or frozen blueberries (not thawed)
- 500 ml (2 cups) grated apples
- 1 Tbsp.
- (15 mL) melted margarine 15 mL (1 tablespoon) lemon juice

Preparation:

1. Put the grill at the centre of the oven. Preheat oven to 180 ° C (350 ° F).
2. In a bowl, mix dry ingredients. Add the margarine and mix until the mixture is just moistened. Book.

3. In a 20-cm (8-inch) square baking pan, combine brown sugar and corn starch. Add the fruits, margarine, lemon juice, and mix well. Cover with crisp and bake between 55 minutes and 1 hour, or until the crisp is golden brown. Serve warm or cold.

Nutritional values:

Calories: 485kcal, Carbohydrates: 85g, Protein: 6 g, Fat: 14 g, Saturated fat:7g, Cholesterol: 30 mg, Sodium: 112 mg, Potassium: 200 mg

111. Raspberry feast meringue with cream diplomat

Ingredients:

Preparation of meringue

- 2 egg whites
- 1/2 cup caster sugar
- 1/4 tsp. vanilla extract
- 1/4 cup crumbled barley sugar

Raspberry mousse preparation

- 1 cup frozen raspberries
- 1/4 cup water
- 2 tbsp. Raspberry Jell-O Powder with No Added Sugar
- 1 1/2 cup Cool Whip
- 1 bowl fresh raspberries

Preparation:

1. To make the meringue, preheat the oven to 350 o F (175 o C) and line a baking sheet with parchment paper.
2. In a blender or bowl, whisk egg whites until the foam is obtained. Gently add the sugar while whisking until you get firm, shiny picks. Stir in vanilla extract and crumbled barley sugar.
3. Shape the meringues on the coated cookie sheet and place in the preheated oven. Turn off the oven and wait 2 hours. Do not open the oven. Once the meringues are dry, break the meringues into small bites.
4. To make the mousse, put frozen raspberries and water in a small saucepan. Heat until raspberries melt and are tender. Put these raspberries in a blender. Add the Jell-O powder and mix. Once the raspberries have completely cooled, incorporate the Cool Whip.
5. To shape the raspberry, place in balloon glasses for individual portions or in a large cake pan first a layer of raspberry mousse, then a layer of meringue, then fresh raspberries. Repeat the layers. Refrigerate for a few hours before serving.

Nutritional values:

Energy: 187kcal, Protein: 8g, Fat: 16g, Carbohydrates: 4g, Dietary fibbers: 5g, Potassium: 199mg, Calcium: 188mg, Phosphate: 170mg

112. Pear crumble with vanilla sauce

Servings: 4

Ingredients:

- 4 pears (150g each)
- 1 tbsp lemon juice
- 100g flour
- 50g sugar
- 80g butter
- 1 teaspoon cinnamon
- For the vanilla sauce:
- 150ml water
- 50ml cream
- 1 packet of vanilla sugar
- 1 teaspoon of vanilla pudding powder

Preparation:

1. For the crumble, knead the cold butter, flour, sugar, and cinnamon and crumble. Chill for 30 minutes.
2. Chop the pears and drizzle with the lemon juice. Pour into a greased baking dish (or 4 small dishes) and spread the crumble over it. Bake in a preheated oven at 180 ° C for about 25 minutes. (For small molds about 20 minutes) For the vanilla sauce, stir all the ingredients with a whisk and bring to the boil while stirring.

Nutritional values:

Energy: 407kcal, Protein: 3g, Potassium: 230mg, Phosphate: 53mg

113. Rice casserole with cherries

Servings 4

Ingredients:

- 300ml water
- 150 ml of cream
- 1 sachet of vanilla sugar

- 100g rice pudding
- 1 egg
- 1 egg white
- 50g butter
- 50g sugar
- 200g sour cherries, preserve drained
- 1 tbsp breadcrumbs
- 1 tablespoon of sugar

Preparation:

1. Mix the water and cream in a saucepan and bring to a boil. Scatter the rice pudding and vanilla sugar and cook for 25 minutes over low heat, stirring occasionally. Let cool down lukewarm.
2. Mix the butter with the sugar until creamy and stir in the egg yolks. Beat the egg whites until stiff. Stir the rice pudding into the fat and fold in the egg whites.
3. Put the cherries in a baking dish and pour in the rice mixture. Sprinkle with sugar and breadcrumbs. Bake at 180 ° C for about 30 minutes.

Nutritional values:

Energy: 426kcal, Protein: 6g, Potassium: 172mg, Phosphate: 97mg

114. Crepes with protein-free flour

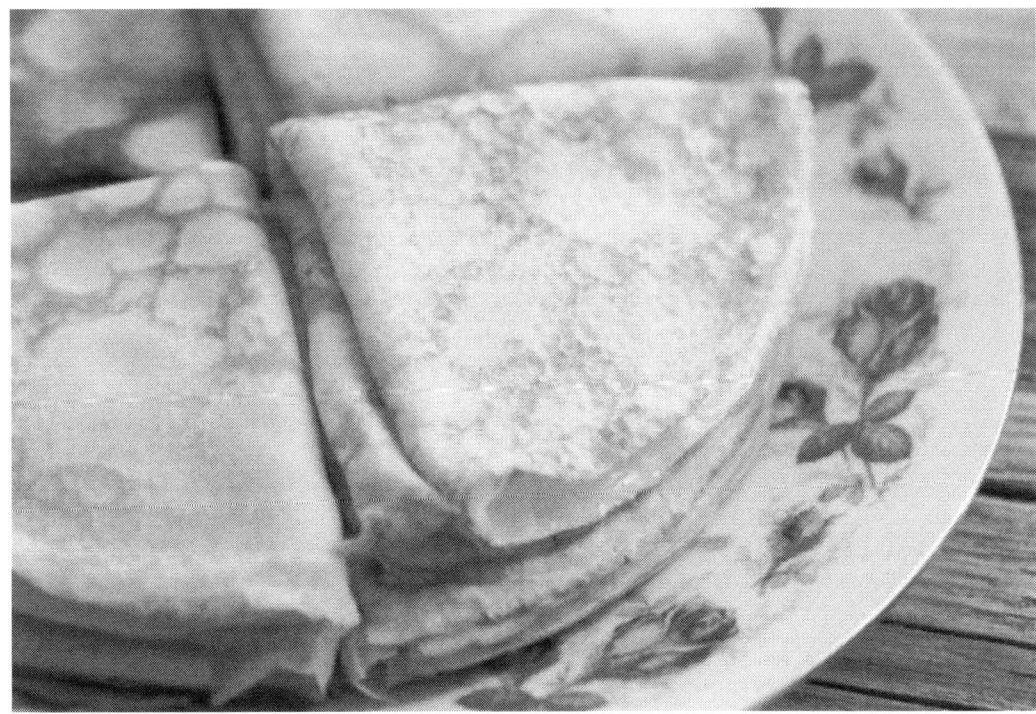

With this dose come about 10-12 crepes

Ingredients:

- Protein-free flour 50 g
- 1egg
- Butter 10 g
- Protein-free milk 125 g
- A pinch of salt

Preparation:

1. In a small pan, melt the butter.
2. Prepare a batter with the egg, milk, and protein-free flour: it must be smooth and homogeneous. Add the melted butter to the batter and mix again to mix everything. Cover with cling film and let it rest for at least 1 hour.
3. Heat a non-stick pan on the fire (diameter of 12-15 cm), and when it is hot, pour a little batter into the centre of the pan and then, tilting and rotating it, try to distribute it over the entire surface. Let the crepe set on one side and then turn it with the help of a spatula. As soon as it is ready, slide it onto a plate.
4. Prepare the rest with the same procedure.

They are excellent. You can fill them with jams and make a dessert or with a salty filling and serve them as a first course.

Nutritional values:

Water: 56 g, Calories/Energy: 410 kcal, Protein: 8 g, Lipids: 18 g, Carbs: 50 g, Sodium: 563 mg, Phosphorous: 161 mg, Potassium: 145mg

115. Wine biscuits with protein-free flour

Servings: 1 - 8

Ingredients:

- Protein-free flour 200 g
- Sugar 80 g + about 30 g to decorate
- Sweet wine like sparkling wine 100 ml
- Corn oil 50 g
- ¼ of a sachet of baking powder for cakes
- Aniseed

Preparation:

1. In a bowl, put the flour, 80 g of sugar, aniseed, oil, and yeast.

2. Add the wine and mix it with a fork. When the liquid is absorbed, put the dough on a surface and finish kneading. With your hands make sticks that you will cut as long as you like.
3. Close them and pass them in the remaining sugar before placing them on the baking sheet. Bake at about 150 ° in a ventilated oven.

Excellent biscuits for breakfast or a snack. Phosphorus and sodium come from the yeast used.

Nutritional values:

Water: 25 g, Calories/Energy: 470kcal, Protein: 1 g, Lipids: 15 g, Carbohydrates: 79 g, Potassium: 73 mg, Sodium: 113 mg, Phosphorous: 152 mg

116. Strawberry tiramisu

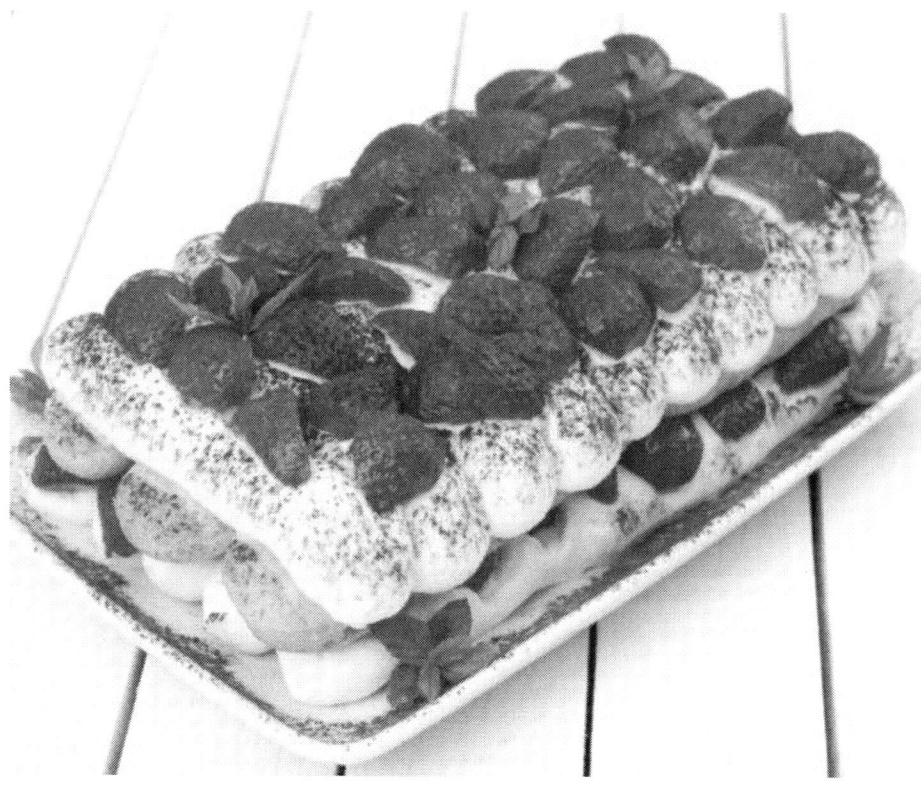

Servings: 4

Ingredients:

- 4 ladyfingers
- 4 tbsp almond syrup or amaretto
- 50g sugar
- 1/2 vanilla pod
- 100g mascarpone
- 200g cream quark
- 1 tbsp chopped pistachios

- 200g strawberries

Preparation:

1. Puree half of the strawberries with 1 tablespoon of sugar and the vanilla pulp. Cut the remaining strawberries into small pieces. Mix the mascarpone and cream quark with the remaining sugar.
2. Break the sponge fingers into pieces and divide them into four glasses. Pour almond syrup over it, then spread the strawberry puree and strawberries on top. Pour in the quark mixture and garnish with a piece of strawberry and the pistachios.
3. Let soak in the refrigerator for an hour.

Nutritional values per serving:

Energy: 315kcal, Protein: 7g, Fat: 21g, Carbohydrates: 24g, Dietary fibbers: 2g, Potassium: 185mg, Calcium: 89mg, Phosphate: 154mg

117. Donut-shaped cake with white icing and coloured sprinkles

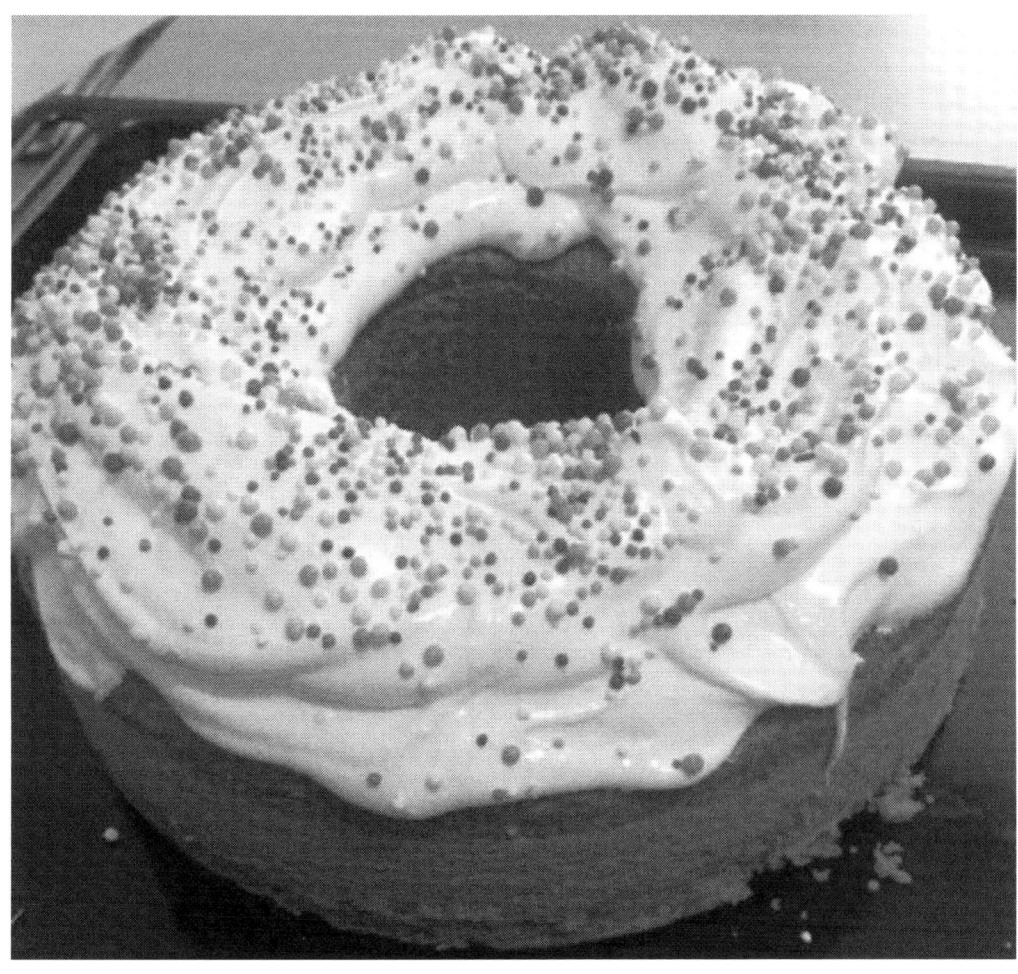

Servings: 10 – 12 people (it is a typical dessert for Easter)

Ingredients:

- Protein-free flour 250 g
- Sugar 75 g
- Lard 100 g
- 1 egg
- Cinnamon
- Grated lemon peel
- Lemon juice
- Alchermes 30 ml
- Half a sachet of baking powder

FOR THE ICING

- 1 egg white
- 60 g of sugar
- Coloured sprinkles

Preparation:

1. On a plane mix flour and yeast.
2. Make a hole in the centre and place the different ingredients: lard, egg, sugar, grated lemon, cinnamon, and lemon juice (these to be measured according to taste).
3. Work quickly: the dough must be soft enough.
4. Divide the dough into 2 parts: a larger one is worked in the shape of a stick, then closed to form a donut. Arrange the dessert on a greased baking sheet (it is fine even if it is placed on parchment paper).
5. With the other smaller part of the dough, make two rolls to be arranged crosswise in the centre of the donut.
6. With scissors, carve the edges of the cake. Bake the dessert in a hot oven at 160 ° -180 ° C.
7. In the meantime, prepare the glaze with the egg white and sugar: it must be very firm, like a meringue.
8. When the cake is freshly baked and still boiling, spread the icing over the dessert with a brush and then decorate with coloured sprinkles.
9. The cake is put back in the warm oven for a few minutes to let the glaze harden.

With the indicated dose came a cake of about 600 g. Calories refer to 100 g.

Nutritional values per serving:

Water: 23 g, Calories/Energy: 409 Kcal, Protein: 2 g, Lipids: 17 g, Potassium: 42 mg, Sodium: 36 mg, Phosphorous: 44 mg

118. Amarena dessert

Servings: 2

Ingredients:

- 100g mascarpone
- 50g sour cream
- 1 packet of vanilla sugar
- 50g Amarena cherries with juice
- 1 tbsp lime juice
- some grated lime zest
- 4 ladyfingers

Preparation:

1. Mix the mascarpone with sour cream, vanilla sugar, lime juice, and zest until creamy. Break the sponge fingers and place them in two dessert bowls. Pour half of the Amarena cherries on top and pour in the cream mixture. Place the remaining Amarena cherries on top.

Nutritional values per serving:

Energy: 360kcal, Protein: 3g, Fat: 25g, Carbohydrates: 31g, Potassium: 132mg, Phosphate: 85mg

119. Peach ice cream

Servings: 4

Ingredients:

- 1 peach (approx. 120g)
- 125 ml of water
- 100g preserving sugar
- 250ml cream

Preparation:

1. Skin the peach and cut into small pieces. Mix with the preserving sugar and water and bring to the boil. Let simmer for a minute. Puree and cool. Whip the cream until stiff and fold into the cold peach mixture. Freeze the mixture, stirring occasionally if possible. Let something thaw before consumption.

Nutritional values per serving:

Energy: 290kcal, Protein: 2g, Fat: 19g, Carbohydrates: 29g, Potassium: 112mg, Phosphate: 44mg

120. Fruit rice

Servings: 4

Ingredients:

- 300ml water
- 200ml cream
- 60g rice pudding
- 30g sugar
- 1 teaspoon vanilla sugar
- 200g fruit cocktail, canned, drained
- 100ml cream, whipped

Preparation:

1. Put the water and cream in a saucepan and bring to a boil. Add the rice pudding while stirring and bring to the boil once. Remove from heat and swell for 40 minutes with the lid closed. Add sugar and vanilla sugar and let cool. Fold in the whipped cream and fruits.

Nutritional values per serving:

Energy: 342kcal, Protein: 3g, Fat: 23g, Carbohydrates: 32g, Dietary fibbers: 1g, Potassium: 148mg, Phosphate: 65mg

121. Tiramisu

Serving 1 - 8

Ingredients:

- 500 g of mascarpone
- 2 whole eggs
- 50 g of sugar
- 1 cup of coffee
- 2 tablespoons of rum
- 12 ladyfingers (about 100 g)

Preparation:

1. Work the egg yolks with the sugar to create a foam, add the mascarpone, and two tablespoons of rum, and work everything to obtain a homogeneous cream. Separately, whip the egg whites. Once the egg whites are perfectly whipped, add them to the mixture of egg yolks, sugar, and mascarpone. Do this gently, mixing from the bottom up, so as not to dismantle the egg whites.

2. In the meantime, you will have prepared and left the coffee to cool. Quickly dip the ladyfingers in the coffee, being careful not to soak them too much because they would fall apart.
3. Distribute the soaked biscuits in a bowl and cover with the mascarpone cream.
4. If you prefer, you can also prepare this dessert in individual portions using rather shallow water glasses.
5. Let it cool in the refrigerator for at least a couple of hours before serving.

** I've eliminated the chocolate and reduced the sugar but it remains one of the most loved desserts. **

Nutritional values:

Protein: 8 g, Calories: 383 kcal, Potassium 4 *, Low Phosphorus, Lipids: 32 g, Cholesterol: 148 mg

122. Fake berry cheesecake

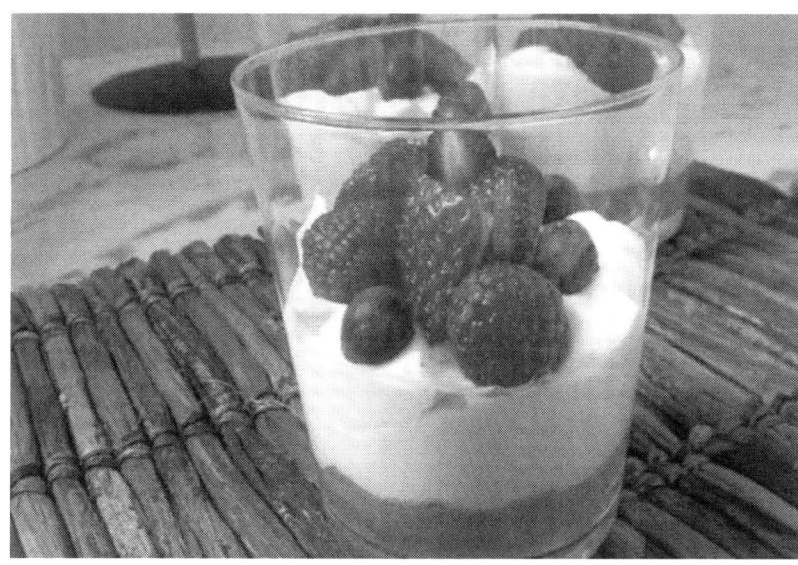

Serving 1 - 4

Ingredients:

- 80 g of dry biscuits (digestive)
- 200 ml of liquid cream
- 150 g of Greek yogurt 0%
- 20 g of butter
- 1 tablespoon of honey
- 100 g of strawberries
- 50 g of raspberries
- 50 g of blueberries

Preparation:

1. Blend the biscuits with the butter and with this mixture prepare the base in 4 glasses.
2. Whip the cream, work the yogurt with the honey and then mix the two ingredients that you will divide into 4 glasses above the biscuit base.
3. Clean the strawberries and berries, cut the strawberries into small pieces (unless they are wild strawberries) and divide the fruit into glasses.
4. Cover each glass with cling film and let it rest in the refrigerator at least 1 hour before serving.

I called it "fake" because in reality there is no "cheese" but 0% Greek yogurt. Furthermore, to maintain the indicated values, I recommend using only the indicated berries: blueberries, raspberries, and strawberries.

Nutritional values:

Protein: 5 g, Calories: 293 kcal, Potassium: 4 *, Low Phosphorus, Lipids: 19 g, Cholesterol: 69 mg

123. Bread cake

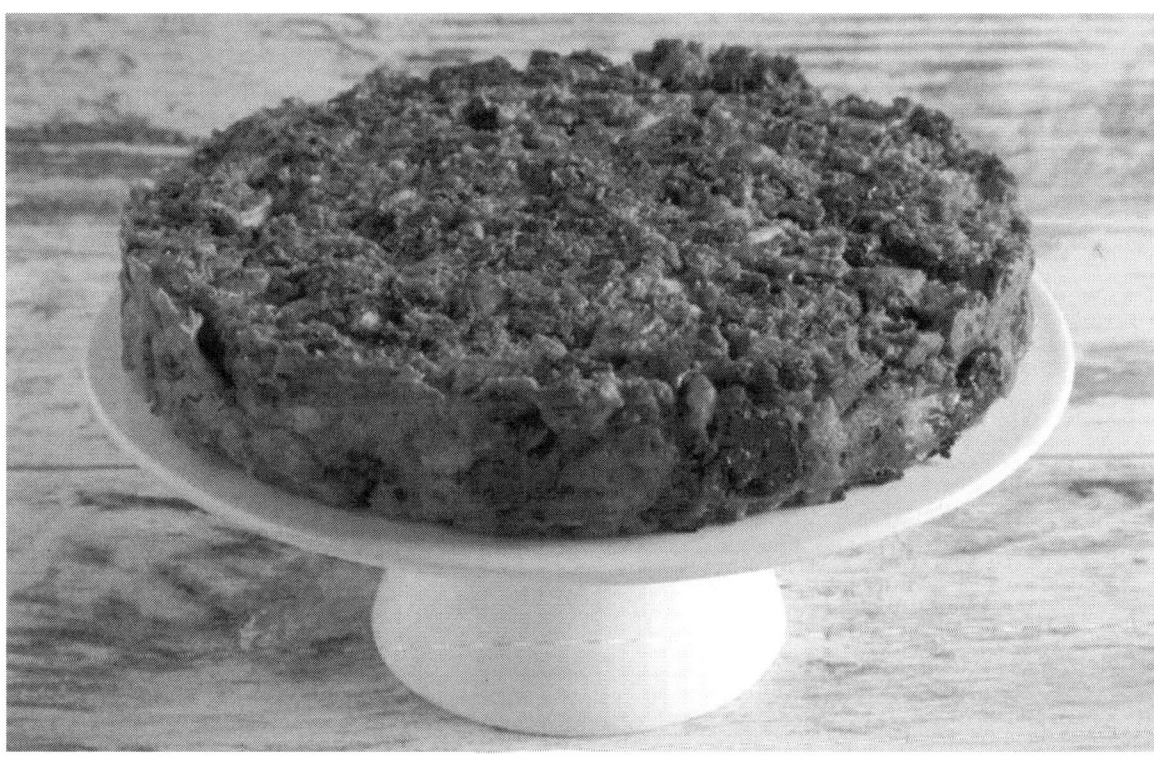

Serving: 6

Ingredients:

- 6 stale rolls (300 g)
- 80 g of sugar
- 3 whole eggs

- 100 g of amaretti biscuits
- 100 g of raisins
- 1 grated lemon
- (zest + lemon juice) (100 g)
- 10 g of cocoa
- 1 handful of pine nuts (15 g)
- 1 litre of whole or semi-skimmed milk

Preparation:

1. Take the sandwiches and dip them in milk for at least 4 hours (the longer they stay in the milk the better).
2. The raisins must be placed in a container with water at least 1 hour before preparation.
3. Place the eggs and the macaroons in a bowl crumbled, lemon juice and zest, raisins, cocoa, sugar and beat everything vigorously. Then add the softened sandwiches and mix everything until you get a mixture homogeneous.
4. Finally, put the dough in the pan (lined with a sheet of parchment paper) and add it over the pine nuts. Bake in the oven at 180 ° for about 1 hour.

This is a high-calorie dessert, with a medium-high content of proteins and glycides. Low lipids, but beware of sugars, they are rapidly absorbed, therefore able to raise triglycerides. The potassium content is very high, dialysis patients should be careful.

Nutritional values per serving:

Calories/Energy: 447 kcal, Protein: 16 g, Lipids: 8 g, Glycides: 82.6 g, Calcium: 260 mg, Sodium: 588 mg, Potassium: 627 mg, Phosphorous: 329 mg

124. Walnut and hazelnut cake

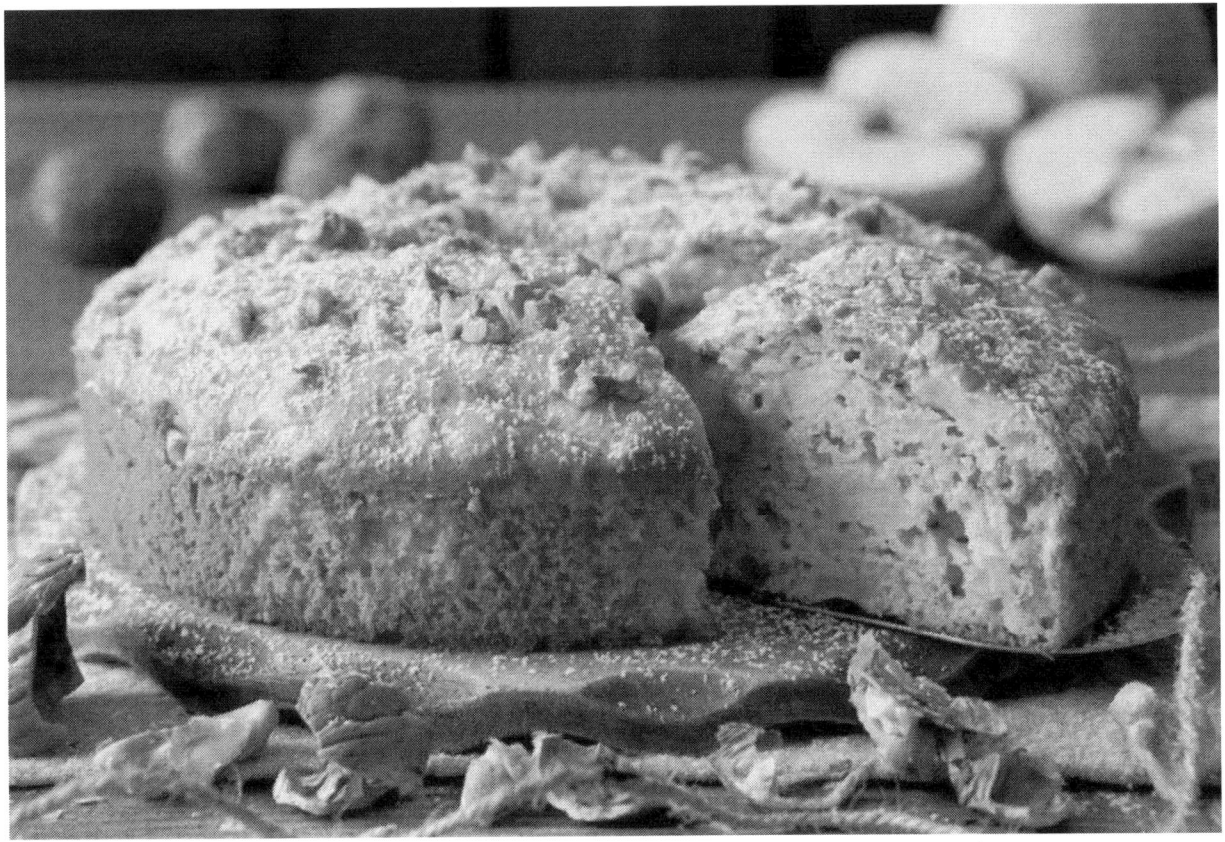

Serving: 8

Ingredients:

- 300 g of wheat flour 00
- 150 g of sugar
- 4 eggs
- 100 g of walnuts (without shell)
- 100 g of hazelnuts
- 1 glass of whole milk
- 1 sachet of vanilla sugar
- 1 sachet of yeast (16 g)
- 120 g of soft butter

Preparation:

1. Put the softened butter and it in a bowl of sugar and work them well with a small whisk
2. until a soft dough is obtained, add a little at a time the eggs (which must previously be beaten with a fork), the flour sifted, baking powder, vanilla sugar, hazelnuts, finely chopped walnuts, and milk.
3. Butter a cake pan and pour the mixture.

4. Bake for 30 minutes at 150 C ° and 30 minutes at 180 C °.

Small calorie bomb with good protein content, which can be reduced if replace normal flour with low-protein flour. Good news for nuts lovers: the reasonable potassium content.

Nutritional values per serving:

Calories/Energy: 531.8 kcal, Protein: 12.5 g, Lipids: 31.6 g, Glycides: 62.8 g, Calcium: 100 mg, Sodium: 56 mg, Potassium: 244 mg, Phosphorous: 205 mg

125. Sandy cake

Serving: 6

Cooking time: 40-50 min., At 180 ° C.

Ingredients:

- 300 g of starch
- 200 g of butter
- 200 g of sugar
- 3 whole eggs
- Half a sachet of yeast (8 g)

Preparation:

1. In a bowl, combine the starch, whole eggs and butter, and sugar.
2. Add the well-dissolved yeast and mix until the mixture becomes uniform.
3. Pour the mixture into the pan and put it in the oven.
4. Cooking time: 40-50 min., At 180 ° C.

Good caloric intake, but pay attention to the lipids they are very tall and of animal origin. Potassium and phosphorus are low.

Nutritional values per serving:

Calories/Energy: 589.1 kcal, Protein: 3.8 g, Lipids: 30.5 g, Glycides: 79.8 g, Calcium: 29 mg, Sodium: 54 mg, Potassium: 203 mg, Phosphorous: 80 mg

126. Pineapple cake

Serving: 6

Ingredients:

FOR THE BASE:

- 100 g of flour
- 2 eggs
- 100 g of sugar

- 8 g of vanilla yeast

FOR THE CREAM:
- 1 whole egg, 1 yolk
- 10 tablespoons of sugar
- 3 tablespoons of flour
- 500 g of semi-skimmed milk
- 250 g pineapple
- 200 g of cream for desserts
- Grated lemon zest

Preparation:

1. To prepare the base of the cake you have to work flour, sugar, yeast until a homogeneous mixture. Bake at 160 degrees for about 15 minutes. After baking, let the cake cool.
2. Meanwhile, prepare the cream. In a saucepan, place on low heat, beat a whole egg, and the yolk with the sugar and flour. Add the milk lukewarm previously brought to a boil with 1/2 grated lemon zest.
3. Cook everything on a slow fire, continuing to stir for about 4-5 minutes.
4. When the base has cooled, cut the part upper (2/3 sup.). Pour on the bottom the pineapple juice (from the can), then put the prepared cream and a layer of cream.
5. Finally, cover them with the mixture obtained from crumbling of the unused part of the cake (the smaller one) combined with the pineapple cut into small pieces.
6. Before serving, the cake must be in the fridge for 2 hours.

This delicious cake is a sweet temptation for those with a sweet tooth. Provides a high caloric, carbohydrate, and lipid intake. The portions are generous. We point out again that potassium is high.

Nutritional values per serving:

Calories/Energy: 422.7 kcal, Protein: 10.3 g, Lipids: 17 g, Glycides: 60.9 g, Calcium: 152 mg, Sodium: 97 mg, Potassium: 371 mg, Phosphorous: 193 mg

127. Lemon cake

Serving: 6

Ingredients:

- 300 g of "00" flour
- 250 g of sugar
- 2 whole eggs
- 100 g of butter
- 2 lemons to grate (30g)

- The juice of 2 lemons
- 150 g of semi-skimmed milk
- 1 sachet of yeast
- 10 g of pine nuts

Preparation:

1. In a bowl, work the butter and sugar well and the 2 egg yolks. Then add the milk and flour (little by little), mixing well with a whisk. Finally add the grated lemon zest, the lemon juice and mix everything until you get a homogeneous mixture.
2. Finally, add the sachet of yeast and the egg whites previously whipped. Roll out the dough into one baking dish and cover with pine nuts.
3. Put in the oven at 180 ° for about 40 minutes.

This is a high-calorie dessert, low in protein and potassium; medium-high the lipid content. Okay for patients with CKD and on dialysis. Just pay attention to the sugars, which are rapidly absorbed.

Nutritional values per serving:

Calories/Energy: 512.7 kcal, Protein: 9.6 g, Lipids: 17.3 g, Glycides: 85 g, Calcium: 53 mg, Sodium: 43 mg, Potassium: 188 mg, Phosphorous: 120 mg

128. Very soft cake

Serving: 8

Cooking time: 40 min. At about temperature moderate.

Ingredients:

- 500 g of flour 00
- 300 g of sugar
- 150 g of butter
- 5 eggs
- The juice and zest of an orange
- A pinch of salt
- 1 sachet of baking powder (16 g)

Preparation:

1. In a bowl, beat the eggs with the sugar, then add the cold and liquefied butter, the salt, the orange juice, and flour. Mix everything mixing with energy.
2. Add the yeast and keep stirring for a few minutes, until the mixture does not become uniform.
3. Pour into a pan and pass in a hot oven.

**This is a cake with good calorific value. Beware of fats in those with cholesterol problems e triglycerides. In people with CKD, we recommend using protein-free flour: in this way the share of proteins. It is also possible to cut down on sugar by using it alone 50 g.*

Nutritional values per serving:

Calories/Energy: 556.2 kcal, Protein: 11.4 g, Lipids: 19.4 g, Glycides: 89.2 g, Calcium: 34 mg, Sodium: 87 mg, Potassium: 163 mg, Phosphorous: 127 mg

CHAPTER THIRTEEN: Snacks, Entrées and Sides

129. Pear crumble with vanilla sauce

Servings: 4

Ingredients:

- 4 pears (150g each)
- 1 tbsp lemon juice
- 100g flour
- 50g sugar
- 80g butter
- 1 teaspoon cinnamon
- For the vanilla sauce:
- 150ml water
- 50ml cream
- 1 packet of vanilla sugar
- 1 teaspoon of vanilla pudding powder

Preparation:

For the crumble, knead the cold butter, flour, sugar, and cinnamon and crumble. Chill for 30 minutes. Chop the pears and drizzle with the lemon juice. Pour into a greased baking dish (or 4 small dishes) and spread the crumble over it. Bake in a preheated oven at 180 ° C for about 25 minutes. (For small molds about 20 minutes) For the vanilla sauce, stir all the ingredients with a whisk and bring to the boil while stirring.

Nutritional values per serving:

Energy: 407kcal, Protein: 3g, Potassium: 230mg, Phosphate: 53mg

130. Rice casserole with cherries

Servings: 4

Ingredients:

- 300ml water
- 150 ml of cream
- 1 sachet of vanilla sugar
- 100g rice pudding
- 1 egg

- 1 egg white
- 50g butter
- 50g sugar
- 200g sour cherries, preserve drained
- 1 tbsp breadcrumbs
- 1 tablespoon of sugar

Preparation:

1. Mix the water and cream in a saucepan and bring to a boil. Scatter the rice pudding and vanilla sugar and cook for 25 minutes over low heat, stirring occasionally. Let cool down lukewarm.
2. Mix the butter with the sugar until creamy and stir in the egg yolks. Beat the egg whites until stiff. Stir the rice pudding into the fat and fold in the egg whites.
3. Put the cherries in a baking dish and pour in the rice mixture. Sprinkle with sugar and breadcrumbs. Bake at 180 ° C for about 30 minutes.

Nutritional values per serving:

Energy: 426kcal, Protein: 6g, Potassium: 172mg, Phosphate: 97mg

131. Tantalizing artichokes

Servings: 6

Ingredients:

- 900 g of artichokes (clean we consider 700 g)
- 60 g of capers
- 6 tablespoons of breadcrumbs
- The juice of 3 lemons
- 3 cloves of garlic
- 5 handfuls of parsley
- 5 bunches of mint
- 8 tablespoons of olive oil
- 10 tablespoons of vinegar
- Pepper as required

Preparation:

The artichokes are cleaned by removing the outer leaves harder and then washed with water acidulated with lemon (to keep them from blackening). They are divided into four parts the hearts and cook them in a pot with oil and garlic; halfway through cooking, adjust the pepper and add a nice sprig of chopped mint, the washed capers, parsley, and 10 tablespoons of vinegar. Before removing from the heat, it is dusted with breadcrumbs.

Note: no salt was added, as the artichokes and capers already contain a lot of sodium. This side dish is low in protein and therefore goes a long way well in people with CKD. The caloric content is low and the lipids are mainly of plant origin. Dialysates need to pay attention to the potassium that is particularly tall.

Nutritional values per serving:

Calories/Energy: 19.8 kcal, Protein: 2 g, Lipids: 0.2 g, Glycides: 2.7 g, Calcium: 100 mg, Sodium: 155 mg, Potassium: 439 mg, Phosphorous: 78 mg

132. Sweet and sour onions

Servings: 6

Ingredients:

- 600 g of spring onions
- 1 tablespoon of sugar
- 6 tablespoons of white vinegar
- 10 tablespoons of olive oil
- Pepper as required

Preparation:

1. Wash the onions well and then blanch them for a few minutes. Then gently cook them in oil and when almost cooked add the pepper, sugar, and vinegar.
2. Leave them to flavour for a few minutes on the fire before serving them at the table.

** This side dish contains very little protein and therefore it works great in patients with advanced CKD, plus it is low in calories, and lipids are contained (to further reduce them use less oil) and therefore it is good for people who need to lose weight. Spring onions have an average potassium content: dialysis patients can enjoy them in complete tranquillity.**

Nutritional values per serving:

Calories/Energy: 35 Kcal, Protein: 1.3 g, Lipids: 0.1 g, Glycides: 7.6 g, Potassium: 230 mg, Calcium: 51 mg, Sodium: 13 mg, Phosphorous: 48 mg

133. Carrot salad

Servings: 4

Ingredients:

- 5 carrots
- The juice of one lemon
- 1 tablespoon of olive oil
- 2 pinches of salt

Preparation:

1. Take the carrots, clean them and wash them. Cut them into strips in a bowl.
2. Season with the juice of lemon, oil, and salt.
3. Serve cold.

dietary dish: low-calorie, low-fat and low protein. The energy contribution provided by this salad is modest.

Nutritional values per serving:

Calories/Energy: 24.7 kcal, Protein: 1.3 g, Fat: 0 g, Calcium: 49 mg, Phosphorous: 42 mg, Sodium: 56 mg, Potassium: 219 mg

134. Tofu patties

Servings: 2 (4 pieces)

Ingredients:

- 160g tofu
- 100g carrots, roughly grated
- 1 onion
- 4 tbsp rapeseed oil
- 2 egg whites
- 2 tbsp wheat flour
- Salt, pepper, cumin

Preparation:

1. Coarsely grate the tofu on a grater. Finely dice the onion and sauté in 1 tablespoon rapeseed oil.
2. Add the carrots and sauté briefly. Let cool down. Mix in the egg white, flour, and tofu and season.

3. Fry the patties in the remaining rapeseed oil.

Nutritional values per serving:

Energy: 306kcal, Protein: 12g, Fat: 24g, Carbohydrates: 11g, Dietary fibbers: 3g, Potassium: 262mg, Calcium: 133mg, Phosphate: 125mg

135. Potato gratin

Servings: 2

Ingredients:

- 300g boiled potatoes, soaked
- 50g leek
- 30g smoked bacon
- 1 cup of creme fraiche with herbs
- 30g Gouda, 48% fat (1 slice)
- 1 tbsp breadcrumbs
- 1 tbsp cold butter

Preparation:

1. Cut the boiled potatoes into slices. Finely dice the bacon and leave it in a pan. Add the finely chopped leek rings and cook until soft. Add creme fraiche and stir well. Mix in the potatoes and pour into a baking dish. Cut the Gouda into small cubes and mix with the breadcrumbs. Sprinkle over the gratin and top with flakes of butter. Bake at 200 ° C for about 20 minutes.

Nutritional values per serving:

Energy: 539kcal, Protein: 9g, Potassium: 409mg, Phosphate: 200mg

136. Cucumber salad, pulled through slowly

Servings: 4

Ingredients:

- 1 cucumber
- 1 tbsp. salt
- 100 ml of water
- 100 ml white wine vinegar
- 2 tbsp. cane sugar
- 5 peppercorns, crushed
- 1/2 teaspoon cinnamon

- 1/2 teaspoon of allspice
- 1 teaspoon chili powder
- 1 teaspoon ginger powder

Preparation:

1. The salad has to brew a day before it is eaten, so start early! Wash the cucumber and cut it into thin slices, put them in a bowl, sprinkle with salt and stir, shake well so that the salt gets everywhere. Then let it steep for half an hour.
2. Meanwhile, in a saucepan, mix water, vinegar, sugar, pepper, cinnamon, allspice, chili, and ginger and bring to the boil once, then let cool again with the lid closed. Rinse the lettuce slices and pour off the water. If necessary, dry in a towel. Add the dressing from the pot to the salad slices and let everything sit in the fridge for a day.

Nutritional values per serving:

Energy: 49kcal, Protein: 1g, Carbohydrates: 5g, Potassium: 234mg, Sodium: 500mg, Calcium: 34mg, Phosphate: 21mg

137. Turnip vegetables

Servings: 2

Ingredients:

- 150g turnip
- 100g potato cubes (watered)
- 100g onion
- 100g pear (canned)
- 100ml vegetable stock
- 1 tbsp rapeseed oil
- 100g creme fraiche
- Salt, marjoram

Preparation:

1. Clean and dice the turnips, dice the onion.
2. First sweat the onion in the oil, then add the diced rutabaga and the diced potatoes.
3. Pour in the broth and cook for 20 minutes.
4. Dice the pear and add.
5. Refine with the creme fraiche and season to taste.

Nutritional values per serving:

Energy: 283kcal, Protein: 3g, Fat: 18g, Carbohydrates: 25g, Dietary fibbers: 6g, Potassium: 430mg, Calcium: 86mg, Phosphate: 100mg

138. Cucumber salad with mint

Servings: 2

Ingredients:

- 300g cucumber peeled and diced
- 1 tbsp yogurt 3.5% fat
- 50ml cream
- 10 mint leaves
- Salt, pepper, piece of garlic
- 1 tbsp olive oil
- 1 teaspoon white balsamic vinegar

Preparation:

1. Put all the ingredients for the sauce in a tall container and mix with a hand blender until the sauce is green.
2. Pour over the cucumber.

Nutritional values per serving:

Energy: 147kcal, Protein: 2g, Fat: 14g, Carbohydrates:4g, Dietary fibbers: 1g, Potassium: 260mg, Calcium: 66mg, Phosphate: 67mg

139. Green beans in salad

Serving: 1

Ingredients:

- 400 gr of green beans

FOR THE DRESSING

- 1 tablespoon of vinegar or lemon juice
- A pinch of salt
- 3 tablespoons of extra virgin olive oil
- 1 tablespoon of chopped parsley

Preparation:

1. Clean the green beans by cutting them off at both ends, wash them well and throw them in 3-4 litres of boiling water. Let them cook for about 10 minutes, then drain and put them in another pot also containing 3-4 litres of lightly salted boiling water. Cook for another 10 minutes, then drain them by passing them in water and ice to keep them crunchy and with a bright colour.
2. Emulsify the ingredients of the dressing in a bowl and add the drained green beans.

As for other vegetable dishes presented, we remind you that double boiling reduces the potassium value by about 1/3.

Nutritional values:

Protein: 2 g, Calories: 87 kcal, Potassium 6 *, Minimum phosphorus, Lipids: 7, Cholesterol: 0 mg

140. Stewed lettuce

Serving: 1 - 4

Ingredients:

- Lettuce salad 400 g
- Spring onions 60 g (heart only)
- Milk 70 g
- 1 teaspoon of starch
- A pinch of salt
- Freshly ground black pepper (optional)

Preparation:

1. Remove the outer leaves of the lettuce heads, wash them in abundant cold water, and cut them in half lengthwise.
2. Slice the spring onions.
3. Arrange the salad and spring onions in a large, low saucepan, cover with the milk in which you have dissolved the teaspoon of starch, add salt.
4. Put the saucepan with the lid on the heat and cook over low heat for about 10 minutes.
5. Serve the salad piping hot with ground pepper.

A different and tasty way to present this vegetable which is usually eaten raw.

Nutritional values:

Protein: 2 g, Calories: 30 kcal, Potassium 7 *, Low Phosphorus, Lipids: 1 g, Cholesterol: 1 mg

141. Gratin onions

Serving: 1 - 4

Ingredients:

- 600 g of Tropea red onions
- 1 sprig of parsley (about 15 g)
- 2 tablespoons of breadcrumbs
- 3 tablespoons of extra virgin olive oil
- A pinch of salt
- A grind of pepper

Preparation:

1. Peel the onions and blanch them whole for 7-8 minutes, drain and divide them in two.
2. Cover a baking sheet with parchment paper and arrange the onions with the cut side facing up, salt and pepper, cover with plenty of chopped parsley, and sprinkle with breadcrumbs. Finish by sprinkling with extra virgin olive oil. Bake at 180 ° C for about 40-50 minutes until the onions are well cooked, wilted, and lightly toasted. If you want to obtain a gratin and golden effect, put the oven in grill mode for a few minutes after cooking.
3. Serve the onions hot.

Few and simple ingredients for a very tasty side dish. Of course, you must love the onions!

Nutritional values:

Protein: 2 g, Calories: 107 kcal, Potassium 5 *, Low Phosphorus, Lipids: 5 g, Cholesterol: 0 mg

142. Zucchini with protein-free bechamel

Serving: 1 - 4

Ingredients:

- 800 gr of small, very fresh courgettes
- A modest pinch of salt
- 2 tablespoons of grated Parmesan cheese
- (FOR THE BECHAMEL)
- 50 g of butter
- 50 g of protein-free flour
- ½ litre of protein-free milk
- 1 small pinch of salt
- 2 tablespoons of grated Parmesan cheese

Preparation:

1. Wash the courgettes well, cut them at both ends, and cook them for 5-6 minutes in 3-4 litres of boiling water. Drain them and immerse them immediately in another saucepan where you have boiled another 3-4 litres of water with salt. Cook for another 5 minutes.
2. Once cooked, cut them in half and arrange them in a baking dish, keeping one aside that you will serve in cubes on top of each portion. Cover with the béchamel and sprinkle with grated cheese. Put them in the oven until the surface is golden.
3. Serve immediately.
4. For the bechamel sauce: heat the butter in a non-stick saucepan and add the flour over a very low heat, stirring quickly so that no lumps form. Add the milk that you have previously heated and, always stirring, cook for about 10 minutes. In the end, off the heat, add the grated cheese, and season with salt.

The use of protein-free flour and milk for the preparation of bechamel makes this dish suitable for a diet with low proteins, where indicated by the doctor. I've also provided for the double boiling of the zucchini to reduce the amount of potassium.

Nutritional values:

Protein: 6 g, Calories: 280 kcal, Potassium 10 *, Medium Phosphorus, Lipids: 18 g, Cholesterol: 40 mg

143. Friselle with cherry tomatoes

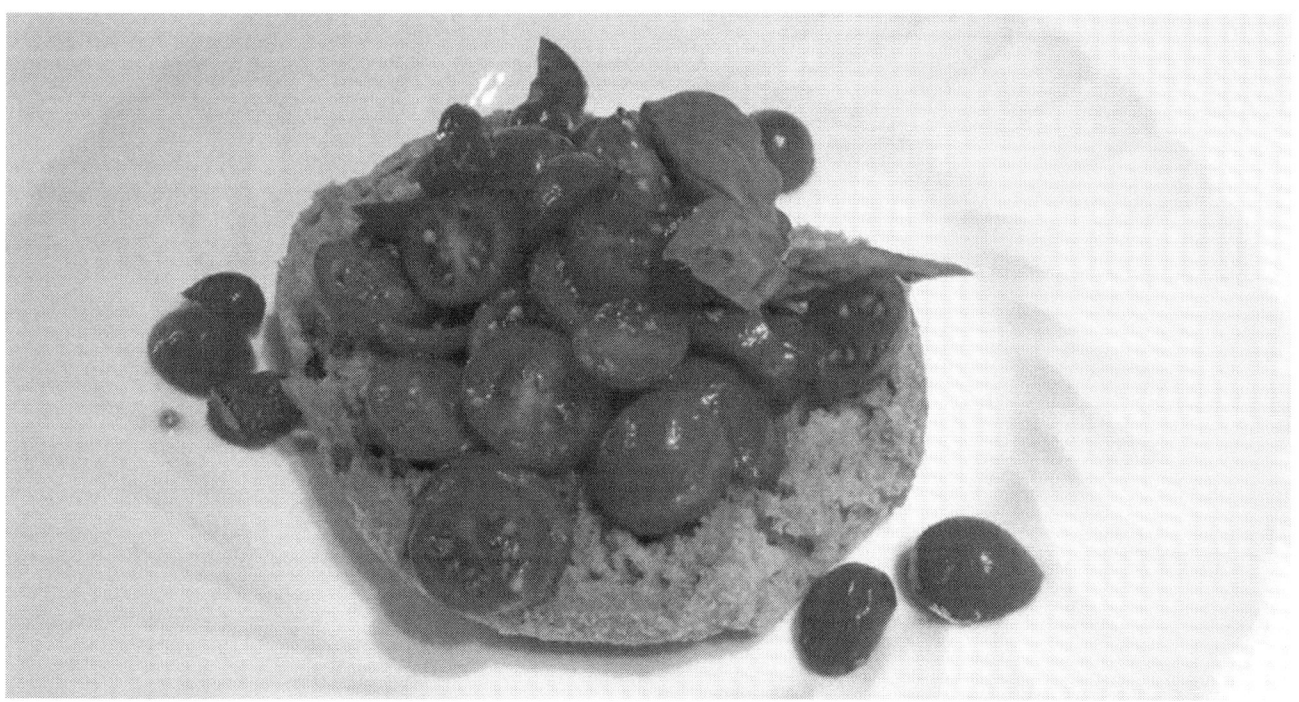

Serving: 1 - 4

Ingredients:

- 4 friselle (about 40 g each)
- 400 g of cherry tomatoes
- 4 tablespoons of extra virgin olive oil
- A few basil leaves
- A handful of dried oregano
- A pinch of salt
- A pinch of red pepper

Preparation:

1. Moisten the friselle by immersing them in a bowl of cold water for a few seconds.
2. Arrange them on a plate and season with a tablespoon of olive oil each. Wash and cut the cherry tomatoes into small pieces and distribute them on the oiled friselle. Season with a pinch of salt, dried oregano, and a few basil leaves.

Summer, fresh and, above all, fast!

Nutritional values:

Protein: 6 g, Calories: 245 kcal, Potassium 9 *, Low Phosphorus, Lipids: 11 g, Cholesterol: 0 mg

144. Crispy polenta

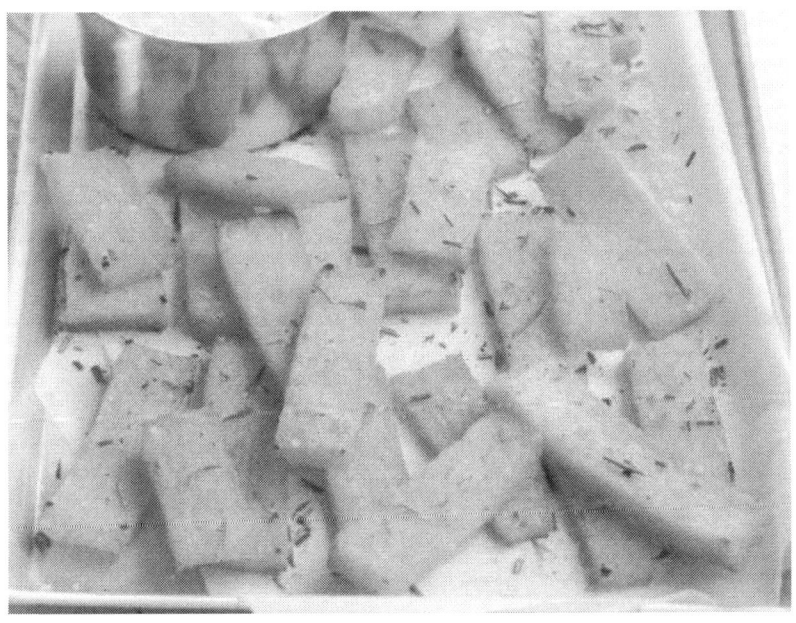

Serving: 4

Ingredients:

- 300 g of polenta flour (precooked)

- 700 ml of water; 200 g of Parmesan cheese
- 2 scant teaspoons of Cervia sea salt
- Pepper
- Breadcrumbs 20 g (1 large spoonful)
- 1 tablespoon of extra virgin olive oil

Preparation:

1. In a non-stick pan with high sides, add the water, salt, oil, and bring to a boil.
2. When it reaches the boiling point, pour the polenta and stir constantly (it must thicken). Transfer the polenta to a baking tray lined with parchment paper and add the parmesan in layers. Spread the breadcrumbs over the entire surface and bake at 200 ° (preheated oven) for 20-25 minutes (monitor cooking).
3. Serve and enjoy according to your imagination.

Tasty single dish. Warning: it is rich in phosphorus so don't forget to take the chelator correctly! Sodium comes from both added salt and Parmesan. Use integral sea salt: it has iodine like iodized salt but has no added potassium!

Nutritional values:

Water: 233 g, Protein: 21 g, Phosphorous: 383 mg, Potassium: 110 mg, Lipids: 18 g, Carbs: 33 g, Sodium: 1266 mg, Calories: 371 kcal

145. "Frattau" bread

Serving: 4

Ingredients:

- Carasau bread 320 g
- Ripe tomatoes 600 g
- Carrot
- Celery
- Onion
- Extra virgin olive oil 20 g
- A few basil leaves
- Salt if allowed
- 4 eggs
- 40 g grated pecorino
- Pepper to taste

Preparation:

1. Prepare the sauce: peel the tomatoes, chop them and place them in a pan with onion, celery and carrot washed and cut into small pieces. Cook for about 20 minutes. Pass with a vegetable mill and over the heat, add the extra virgin olive oil and perfume with a few chopped basil leaves.
2. Boil 2 pots with water: one larger and one smaller. Add a pinch of salt to each of the two pots.
3. In the large, when serving, wet the carasau bread by dipping it with a skimmer in boiling water for a few seconds. Drain, put on the plate, and season in layers with the prepared sauce and cheese.
4. In the saucepan, cook the poached eggs (preferably one at a time). Bring water to a boil and add a tablespoon of vinegar. Lower the heat so that the water only quivers and with the help of a spoon stir the water so that a "vortex" is created in which to slide the eggs. The trick is to be able to "wrap" the egg white around the yolk, preventing the eggs from breaking.
5. Cook for 3 minutes, drain with a slotted spoon and place them in the centre of the plate, on top of the prepared bread.
6. If you like, add the black pepper.

For those in dialysis: it's a single dish and is rich in potassium and phosphorus. Therefore, it is good not to eat the side dish: the tomato sauce is enough! In the following meal, it is better to choose a second course based on meat. For the phosphorus, however, you could not add the pecorino ... or DON'T forget the chelator! Finally, it would be advisable not to add salt to the sauce and water. Just the one contained in carasau bread and pecorino cheese!

Nutritional values:

Water: 274 g, Protein: 22 g, Phosphorous: 338 mg, Potassium: 686 mg, Lipids: 15 g, Carbs: 67 g, Sodium: 460 mg, Calories: 495 kcal

CHAPTER FOURTEEN: Spreads, Dips, Appetizers and Sauces

146. Salmon Cream Cheese

Servings: 10

Ingredients:

- 250g plain cream cheese, double cream level
- 100g fresh cucumber
- 50g smoked salmon
- 1 tbsp. dill chopped
- 1 teaspoon lemon juice
- black pepper

Preparation:

1. Peel the cucumber, remove the seeds and grate coarsely.
2. Finely dice the salmon and mix with the other ingredients.

Nutritional values per serving:

Energy: 93kcal, Protein: 4g, Fat: 8g, Carbohydrates: 1g, Potassium: 55mg, Calcium: 25mg, Phosphate: 52mg

147. Spicy spread

Servings: about 20 servings

Ingredients:

- 100g butter
- 100g tomato paste
- 200g grated carrots
- 2 cloves of garlic
- 1 onion
- 2 tbsp. Italian herbs (frozen)

Preparation:

1. Melt butter in a saucepan, chop onion and garlic, and fry.
2. Also, add the carrots and steam them a little soft so that you can puree them afterward, takes about 5 minutes.

3. Remove from heat and add tomato paste and herbs. Puree and keep in the refrigerator.

Nutritional values per serving:

Energy: 44kcal, Protein: 0g, Fat: 4g, Carbohydrates: 1g, Potassium: 80mg, Sodium: 14mg, Calcium: 9mg, Phosphate: 12mg

148. Bulgur spread

Servings: 15

Ingredients:

- 100ml vegetable stock
- 50g bulgur
- 100g mushrooms
- 1 tbsp rapeseed oil
- 75g margarine
- Salt, pepper, thyme

Preparation:

1. Bring the vegetable stock to the boil and let the bulgur soak in it.
2. Cut the mushrooms into small cubes and steam them in the sunflower oil for a minute.
3. Let both cool and puree salt, pepper, and thyme together with margarine.

Nutritional values per serving:

Energy: 46kcal, Protein: 0g, Fat: 4g, Carbohydrates: 2g, Potassium: 29mg, Phosphate: 17mg

149. Apple and onion lard

Servings: 2

Ingredients:

- 250g diced onions
- 8 tbsp sunflower oil
- 1 apple
- 100g margarine
- Salt pepper
- 1 teaspoon herbs of Provence

Preparation:

1. Steam the onions in the oil until translucent.
2. Peel the apple and grate it finely.

3. Add to the onions and sauté briefly.
4. Season with salt, pepper, and herbs from Provence and let cool.
5. Stir the margarine until creamy and stir in the cooled onion mixture.

Nutritional values per serving:

Energy: 52kcal, Protein: 0g, Fat: 5g, Carbohydrates: 1g, Potassium: 18mg, Phosphate: 5mg

150. Zucchini spread

Servings: 2

Ingredients:

- 250 g zucchini
- 60 g double cream cheese with herbs
- 3 tbsp. olive oil
- 1 tbsp. lemon juice
- Salt pepper

Preparation:

1. Wash and clean the zucchini and cut once lengthways.
2. Place the cut side on a greased baking sheet and bake for about 15 minutes at 200 ° C.
3. Remove the zucchini from the oven, let cool down briefly and cut into cubes.
4. Put the zucchini, cheese, oil, juice, and spices in a tall container and puree with the blender.

Nutritional values per serving:

Energy: 51kcal, Protein: 1g, Fat: 5g, Carbohydrates: 1g, Potassium: 50mg, Sodium: 211mg, Calcium: 15mg

151. Vegetable spread

Servings: 2

Ingredients:

- 100g butter
- 50g chopped onion
- 50g carrots, diced
- 50g zucchini, diced
- 50g red peppers, diced
- Herbal salt, pepper

Preparation:

1. Heat 1 teaspoon of butter in a saucepan and fry the diced vegetables until soft.
2. Season with herb salt and pepper and let cool.
3. Mix the remaining butter with the mixer until creamy and stir in the diced vegetables.

Nutritional values per serving:

Energy: 52kcal, Protein: 0g, Fat: 5g, Carbohydrates: 28g, Potassium: 28mg, Phosphate: 6mg

152. Herbal Cupcakes

Servings: 12 pieces

Ingredients:

- 200g flour
- 2 teaspoons of baking soda
- 1 egg
- 150g low-fat quark
- 2 tbsp. olive oil
- 2 tbsp. chopped parsley
- pinch of salt
- 1 onion
- For the topping
- 200g low-fat quark
- 1 tbsp. chives rolls
- 1 tbsp. chopped parsley
- 100g cream cheese, double cream setting
- Salt pepper

Preparation:

1. Finely chop the onion and sauté in the olive oil until translucent. Let cool.
2. Mix with all other ingredients for the dough with the mixer and divide into 12 muffin cases. Bake at 180 ° C (fan oven 160 ° C) for about 20 minutes.
3. Mix the quark with the cream cheese, herbs, and spices and spread over the muffins.

Nutritional values per serving:

Energy: 121kcal, Protein: 6g, Fat: 5g, Carbohydrates: 13g, Dietary fibbers: 1g, Potassium: 75mg, Calcium: 53mg

153. Salmon cream cheese

Servings: 10

Ingredients:

- 250g plain cream cheese, double cream level
- 100g fresh cucumber
- 50g smoked salmon
- 1 tbsp dill chopped
- 1 teaspoon lemon juice
- black pepper

Preparation:

Peel the cucumber, remove the seeds and grate coarsely. Finely dice the salmon and mix with the other ingredients.

Nutritional values per serving:

Energy: 93kcal, Protein: 4g, Fat: 8g, Carbohydrates: 1g, Potassium: 55mg, Calcium: 25mg

154. Cold cucumber soup

Servings: 2 servings

Ingredients:

- 200g cucumber
- 300ml vegetable stock
- Piece of garlic (to taste)
- 100g creme fraiche
- Salt pepper
- 1 tbsp. white wine vinegar
- 1 tbsp. olive oil
- 1 teaspoon chopped parsley
- 1/2 tomato, diced

Preparation:

Finely grate the cucumber in half. Cut the other half into small pieces and puree with the vegetable stock, garlic, spices, vinegar, and creme fraiche. Add the grated cucumber. Serve well chilled with the diced tomatoes and chopped parsley.

155. Thick cream of carrots (Crecy potage) with protein-free croutons

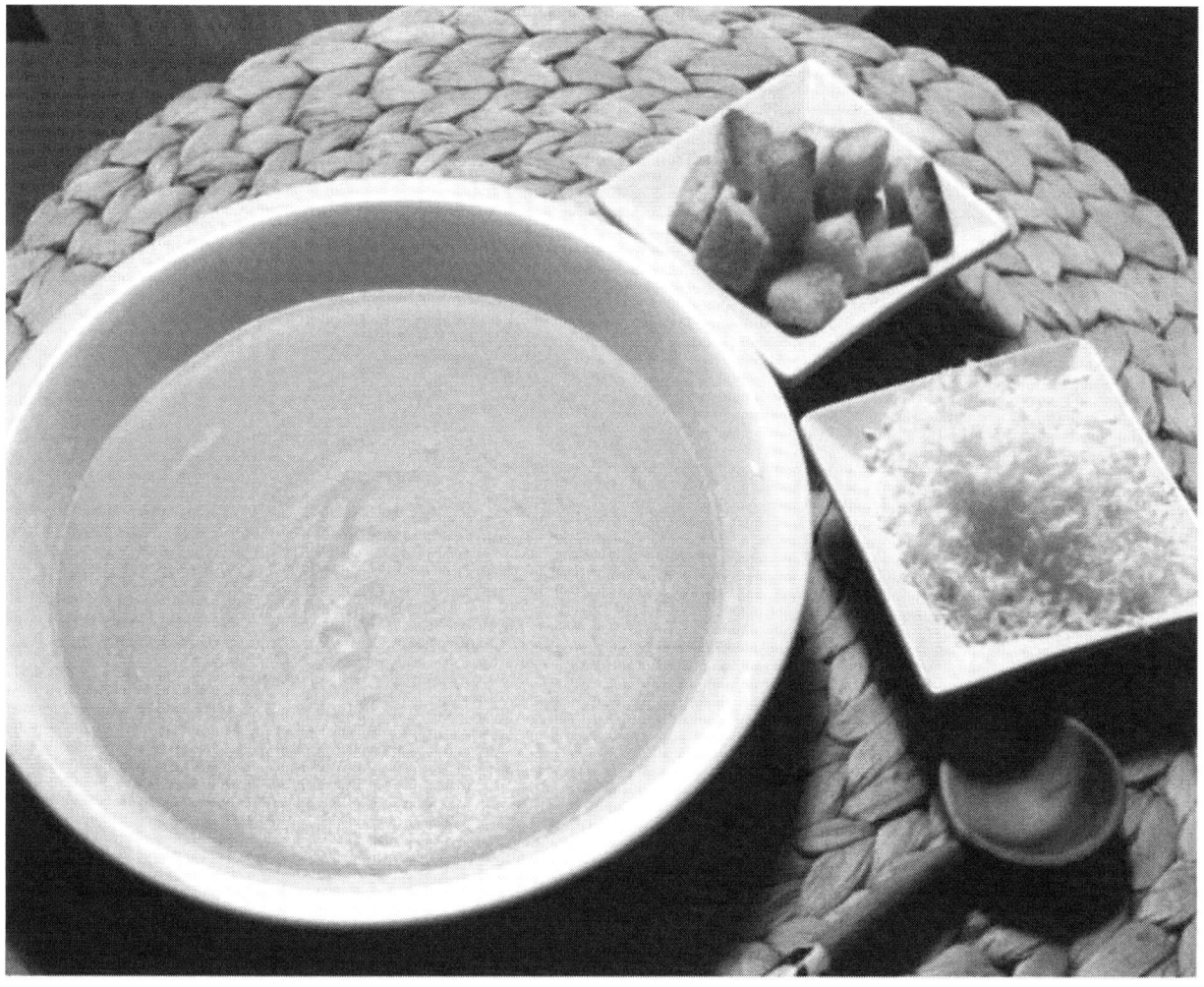

Servings: 1 – 4 (with low-protein bread)

Ingredients:

- 350 grams of peeled carrots
- 50 gr of onion
- 50 gr of rice for soups
- 20 gr of butter
- 2 tablespoons of extra virgin olive oil
- 20 gr of grated Parmesan cheese
- A modest pinch of salt
- (TO ACCOMPANY)
- 4 slices of protein-free bread, without crust, diced and toasted
- 20 gr of grated Parmesan cheese

Preparation:

1. Scrape the carrots, wash them well, cut them into slices, and put them on the stove with 3-4 litres of cold water. Let them boil for 10 minutes, then drain them.
2. Separately, chop the onion and brown it in a saucepan with oil and butter, then add the previously boiled carrots and leave them to flavour for a few minutes, stirring them. Then add about 1 litre of hot water, bring it to the boil again, and then throw the rice into it, letting it cook for about half an hour.
3. Then pass the soup through a vegetable mill or blend it, to make it creamy.
4. When ready to serve, heat the cream obtained, adjust, if necessary, its density (adding a little water), flavour it with Parmesan and salt (a little).
5. Serve hot accompanied by croutons of toasted bread (arranged in a bowl) and grated Parmesan.

The use of protein-free bread for croutons allows you to reduce the value of proteins. A bit of history on the origin of the name: The Battle of Crecy was one of the most important of the Hundred Years War. Beyond the Channel, eating a Crecy soup means commemorating this famous and dramatic battle, in France, it means tasting the best carrots in the country, precisely those from Crecy, in Picardy, cooked with a tasty and comforting recipe.

Nutritional values:

Protein: 5 g, Calories: 238 kcal, Potassium 5 *, Low Phosphorus, Lipids: 13 g, Cholesterol: 22 mg

156. Pumpkin cream with prawns and quinoa

Servings: 1 – 4

Ingredients:

- 300 g of pumpkin pulp
- 8 shrimp, about 100 g
- 2 boiled chestnuts, about 10 g
- 60 g of quinoa
- 20 g of extra virgin olive oil
- 20 g of Greek yogurt 0%
- A pinch of salt

Preparation:

1. Cook the boiled quinoa following the package instructions (each brand can have different times and methods) and let it cool. Spread it on a sheet of parchment paper, cover it with another sheet of parchment paper and roll it out in a thin layer using a rolling pin. Remove the top

sheet of parchment paper and transfer it to a plate. Bake for about 20 minutes at 170 °, until a crunchy layer is formed which you will delicately break up into crackers.

2. Cut the pumpkin into cubes and brown it with a drizzle of oil for a couple of minutes, cover with a little water and cook for another 15 minutes. Turn off and blend in cream.
3. Shell the prawns and sauté them in a pan with a drizzle of oil for 1 minute.
4. Spread the pumpkin cream on each plate, complete with two prawns each, a quinoa cracker, a teaspoon of Greek yogurt, a slice of boiled chestnut, and a drizzle of oil.

Quinoa has a high protein content and is therefore proposed in this recipe only in the form of "crackers" accompanied by pumpkin cream.

Nutritional values:

Protein: 7 g, Calories: 138 kcal, Potassium 6 *, Medium Phosphorus, Lipids: 6 g, Cholesterol: 38 mg

157. Provençal pie with low-protein artichokes

Servings: 1 – 8

Ingredients:

- (FOR THE SHORTCRUST PASTRY)
- 200 gr of protein-free flour
- 100 gr of butter
- 4 tablespoons of water
- ½ teaspoon of salt
- A pinch of salt
- (FOR THE STUFFING)
- 4 artichokes, of the tip type, carefully cleaned (about 300 g)
- ½ lemon
- 30 gr of butter
- 3 whole eggs
- 1 dl of protein-free milk
- 50 gr of grated Gruyere cheese
- 1 small pinch of salt
- 1 pinch of nutmeg
- Freshly ground black pepper

Preparation:

1. The shortcrust pastry: sift the flour and mix it with the diced butter, adding the water and salt. You can do this either manually or with a mixer. Shape into a ball and let it rest covered in a

cool place for at least half an hour. Then roll it out thinly with a rolling pin and line a pan both on the bottom and on the edges. Prick the bottom of the dough with a fork and bake it covered with parchment paper on which you have placed some dried legumes or small ceramic balls (or stones) to proceed to cook in white. Bake at 180 degrees for 15 minutes, then remove the weights and parchment paper.
2. In the meantime, you will have prepared the filling. Clean the artichokes, wash them in water and lemon and boil them for 10 minutes. Drain them, cut them into slices lengthwise, and pass them in the butter for another 5-10 minutes. Carefully arrange them on the bottom of the pan with the previously cooked pasta and then pour over the beaten eggs with the milk, cheese, salt, pepper, and nutmeg.
3. Put the cake in the preheated oven at 180 ° and bake for about 30-40 minutes, until it is well coloured.

*When the nephrologist prescribes it, protein-free products can be used to reduce the intake of proteins. This is the low-protein version of the artichoke pie. The use of protein-free flour and milk does not involve particular recommendations. The brisè dough may be more "floury" at first, but it will compact easily after the first manipulations.**

Nutritional values:

Protein: 6 g, Calories: 279 kcal, Potassium 4 *, Low Phosphorus, Lipids: 18 g, Cholesterol: 130 mg

158. Gratin Scallops

Servings: 1 – 2

Ingredients:

- 4 scallops (the weight of the edible part is about 100g, 25g / each)
- 10 g of butter
- 2 tablespoons of extra virgin olive oil
- 1 clove of garlic and a small sprig of parsley (10 g chopped)
- 1 tablespoon of breadcrumbs
- 2 tablespoons of cognac
- Salt and pepper

Preparation:

1. Wash the scallops, dry them, and put them back in their shells. Place them on an aluminium-coated baking sheet.
2. To prepare the dressing: chop the parsley with the garlic, put the mince in a saucepan with the butter and oil, and as soon as it starts to fry wet with the cognac and "inflamed" to remove the

alcoholic part. You can do this by passing a lighted match over the saucepan immediately after pouring the cognac or by tilting the saucepan slightly towards the gas flame. Be careful to have enough space above the stove to allow the flame to develop without causing damage!

3. At this point, lightly salt and pepper each scallop, pour a spoonful of seasoning and a light sprinkling of breadcrumbs on each one, and put in a preheated oven at 220 ° for about 10 minutes (no more). You can activate the grill for the last two minutes. Serve immediately.

*Although the high sodium content makes scallops a poorly recommended food in diets for those suffering from hypertension, I decided to present a recipe to be reserved for a particular occasion...**

Nutritional values:

Protein: 7 g, Calories: 198 kcal, Potassium 2 *, Medium Phosphorus, Lipids: 14 g, Cholesterol: 25 mg

159. Red onion tart with protein-free flour

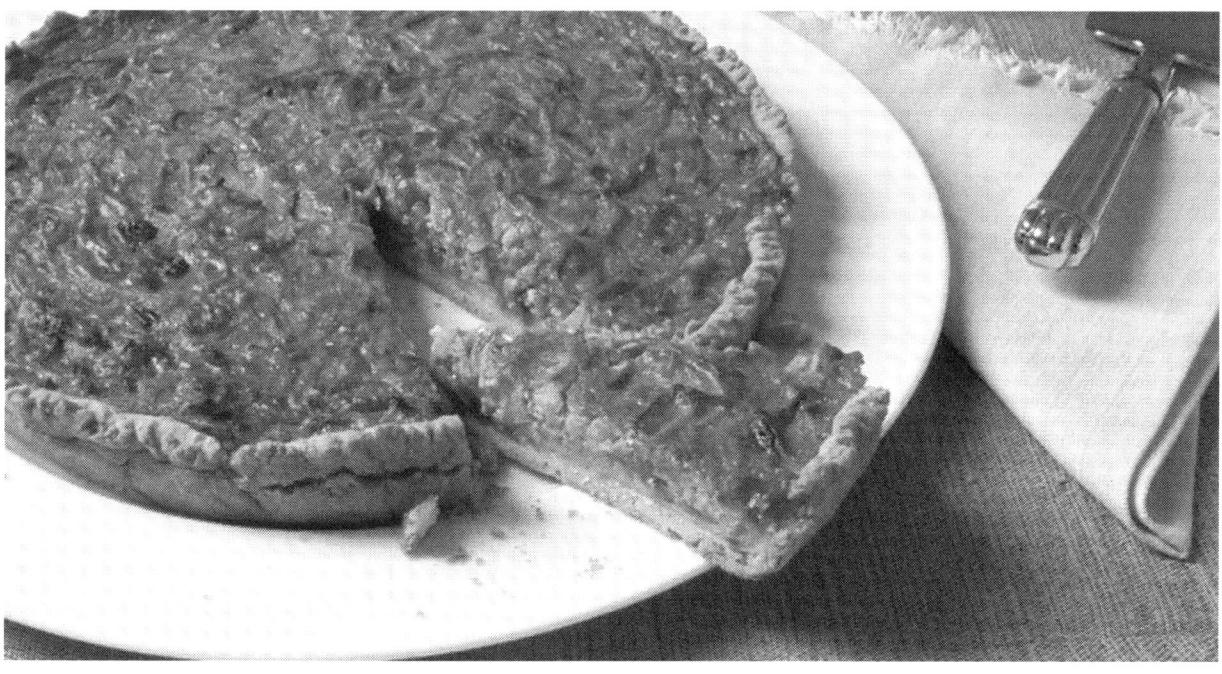

Servings: 1 – 10

Ingredients:

- 600 g of red onions
- 3 tablespoons of extra virgin olive oil
- 2 eggs
- 80 ml of liquid cream
- 30 g of grated Grana Padano
- A pinch of salt
- A grind of pepper

- A spoonful of breadcrumbs
- (FOR THE SHORTCRUST PASTRY)
- 200 g of protein-free flour
- 80 g of butter
- 1 egg
- A modest pinch of salt
- A spoonful of water

Preparation:

1. Prepare the shortcrust pastry, which you will leave to rest in the refrigerator for at least half an hour. Mix the flour with the soft butter, the egg, a drop of water, and a small pinch of salt. Form a ball, wrap it in parchment paper and place it in the refrigerator.
2. Peel the onions and slice them thinly, then put them in a large saucepan with the oil. With the heat to low let them simmer very slowly until they are well wilted. Remove from the heat and let it cool.
3. In a large bowl, beat the eggs with an electric whisk until they are swollen and frothy, add the warm onions, cream, grated parmesan, a pinch of salt, and a pinch of pepper. Mix everything gently to obtain a homogeneous mixture.
4. Line a baking tray, 24 cm in diameter, with parchment paper, roll out the shortcrust pastry, which you have flattened with a rolling pin, prick the bottom, and sprinkle with a spoonful of breadcrumbs. Pour the mixture inside, level the edges with a fork, and bake at 190 ° C for about 50 minutes. For the first 30 minutes cover the pan with a sheet of parchment paper or aluminium which you will remove for the next cooking time.
5. Remove the tart from the oven and let it cool completely before serving, cut into slices.

This tasty tart is perfect as an appetizer or served during an aperitif; it is so good that no one will notice the protein-free flour!

Nutritional values:

Protein: 4 g, Calories: 218 kcal, Potassium 3 *, Low Phosphorus, Lipids: 13 g, Cholesterol: 86 mg

160. Carrot flans with green sauce

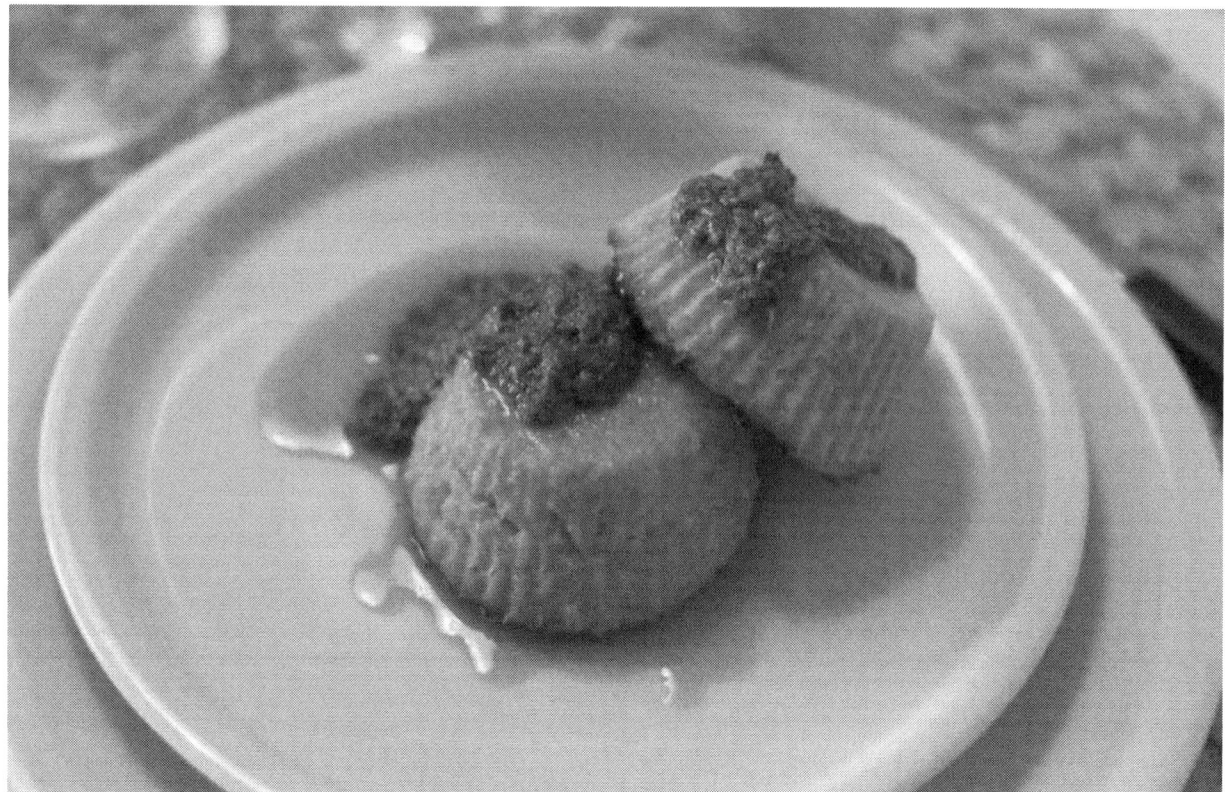

Servings: 1 – 4

Ingredients:

- 500 g of clean carrots
- 2 slices protein-free bread (without crust)
- 1 egg
- 2 tablespoons of grated Parmesan cheese
- 1 pinch of salt
- Butter to grease the molds

FOR THE GREEN SAUCE

- Parsley 25 g
- 1 slice of protein-free bread (without crust)
- 1 modest pinch of salt
- Extra virgin olive oil 50 g
- Vinegar to taste

Preparation:

1. Wash and peel the carrots then proceed to the double boil making them cook for 10 minutes and then another 10-15 minutes until completely cooked.
2. Once cooked, put the carrots in the mixer and blend them with the egg, the bread, the parmesan, and a pinch of salt.
3. Grease 4 molds, with a diameter of 5 cm, and fill them with the blended mixture (if you have silicone molds, very comfortable, you can do without buttering them).
4. Bake in a "bain-marie" for about 25 minutes at 190 °.
5. For the green sauce: soak the slice of bread in the vinegar and then blend it with the parsley adding enough oil and a pinch of salt.
6. Serve the flan warm garnished with a spoonful of green sauce.

A very simple green sauce that goes perfectly and manages to make carrots taste even to those who usually wrinkle their nose in front of this vegetable! Also, for this preparation, the double boiling of the carrots allows to reduce the potassium value by about one third, thus bringing it to 5 * per portion.

Nutritional values:

Protein: 5 g, Calories: 218 kcal, Potassium 7 *, Low Phosphorus, Lipids: 16 g, Cholesterol: 60 mg

CHAPTER FIFTEEN: Fish and Seafood Recipes

161. Rissole of dried codfish or codfish pancakes

Servings: 2

Ingredients:

- 2 lbs. (1/2 - 1kg) cod
- 2 small onions, chopped
- 3 cups (450g) breadcrumbs
- ¼ tsp. (1 ml) black pepper
- 1/4 cup (60g) butter for cooking

Preparation:

Cut the cod into pieces and mix the onions, breadcrumbs, and pepper with them in a bowl. Pass a meat grinder or food processor through the mixture. With the mixture, form pancakes. You should have about 18 fish cakes if you make patties three inches in diameter and 1/2-inch-thick with 2 pounds of fish. For 5 minutes on each side, fry the patties in butter.

Nutrient Analysis:

Energy: 93 g, Protein: 12.3 g, Carbohydrates: 5.1 g, fibbers: 0.7 g, Total fat: 2.9 g, Phosphorus: 139.35 mg, Sodium: 82.7 mg, Potassium: 243.58 mg

162. Steamed Jamaican Fish

Serving 4

Ingredients:

- 4 tilapia fillets (100 g each fillet)
- 1/2 cup (125 mL) olive oil
- 3/4 cup (175 mL) red and green peppers, sliced
- 1/2 cup (125 mL) onion, minced
- 1 / 4 c. teaspoon black pepper
- 1 tbsp. teaspoon chili sauce
- 1 sprig of thyme
- 1 tsp. tablespoon Ketchup
- Juice of 1/2 lime (1 tablespoon lime juice)
- 1 cup hot water

Preparation:

1. Over medium heat, heat the oil in a pan and sauté the onion and peppers.
2. Add the pepper, thyme, ketchup, hot pepper sauce, and lime juice, and 1/2 cup of hot water. Mix thoroughly.
3. In the pan, place the fish and add 1/2 cup of hot water. Use a spoon to coat the fish with sauce and vegetables.
4. Cover and cook in the pan for 5 minutes. Flip the fish, cover, and cook for an extra 5 minutes or until the fish is fully cooked.

Nutrient Analysis:

Energy: 376 g, Protein: 21 g, Carbohydrates: 6 g, fibbers: 1 g, Total Fat: 31 g, Sodium: 106 mg, Phosphorus: 188 mg, Potassium: 432 mg

163. Shrimp and apple stir-fry

Servings: 4

Ingredients:

- ½ lb (227 g) headless shrimp with their shell
- ¾ apple (diced)
- 2 stalks of celery (diced)
- ½ red pepper (small, diced)
- 2 tbsp. 1 tbsp (30 mL) vegetable oil

Marinade

- 1/2 tsp. (2.5 mL) low sodium soy sauce
- 1 tsp. (5 mL) corn-starch
- Pinch white pepper

Sauce

- 1/2 tsp. (2.5 mL) low sodium soy sauce
- 1 tsp. (5 mL) sugar
- 1 tsp. (5 mL) corn-starch
- 2 tsp. 1 tbsp (30 mL) cold water

Preparation:

1. Remove and devein the shrimp shell. Marinate the shrimp for 30 minutes with the marinade ingredients listed above.
2. In a small bowl, combine the ingredients for the sauce, mix well, and set aside.

3. In a non-stick wok, heat about 1 tablespoon of oil and sauté the shrimp until they turn pink. Have them removed from the wok.
4. About 1 Tsp of heat. Oil in a non-adhesive wok. Briefly sauté the celery, then add the diced apple and red pepper, stirring until just finished. Add the shrimp and sauce and stir until the sauce thickens constantly. Serve.

Nutritional values:

Power: 152 g, Protein: 12 g, Carbohydrates: 8 g, fibbers: 1 g, Phosphorus: 130 mg, Potassium: 219 mg, Total Fat: 8 g, sodium: 151 mg.

164. Spicy shrimp linguine

Serving: 4

Ingredients:

- 12 shrimp of size 31/40 (you can also use 6oz of chicken breast cut into small pieces)
- 1 tbsp.
- 1 tbsp canola oil -1 small clove of minced garlic
- 1 pepperoncini or marinated jalapeño pepper
- ¼ cup prepared salsa (mild, medium, or spicy, your choice)
- ¼ cup table cream at 10 %
- 2 cups linguine (or other pasta of your choice), cooked
- ¼ cup chopped cilantro

Preparation:

1. Cook pasta according to the directions for the package.
2. In a medium skillet over medium-high heat, sauté the shrimp in the oil while the pasta is cooking.
3. Add the garlic, pepperoncini, and the prepared salsa when the shrimp starts pulling on the orange-pink colour.
4. Continue to cook over low heat until the shrimp is fully cooked.
5. Turn the heat off when the pasta is ready, and add the cream and pasta to the shrimp mixture. Mix well with the sauce to coat the pasta.
6. Add fresh cilantro to the garnish and serve.

Nutritional values:

Energy: 381 g, Proteins: 16.5 g, Carbohydrates: 50 g, Total Fat: 12 g, Sodium: 464 mg, Phosphorus: 174 mg, Potassium: 297 mg

165. Spaghetti with shrimps

Serving 2

Ingredients:

- 1/2 lb spaghetti or spaghetti
- 1/3 cup extra virgin olive oil
- 1/3 cup dry white wine
- 2 garlic cloves, crushed
- 1/4 tsp. 1 tsp crushed red chili
- pepper 1 red pepper, diced
- 1 lb raw shrimp
- 1/3 cup fresh toasted bread crumbs
- Freshly ground pepper
- Fresh chopped parsley (optional)

Preparation:

1. Cook pasta according to the directions for the package.
2. Heat the oil over medium-low heat in a large skillet and add the garlic and chili pepper. For 1 minute, cook, taking care to stir.
3. Add the pepper and cook (do not brown) for a further 5 minutes. Add the shrimp and cook for an additional 1 minute. Stir in the wine, and then cook over medium heat. Simmer until you see the shrimp turn opaque and start twisting. Keep the sauce warm over low heat if the spaghetti is not ready.
4. Drain the pasta in a large dish and place it in it. Pour the pasta over the sauce, add the bread crumbs and toss to coat the pasta.
5. Use freshly ground black pepper and parsley to serve.

Nutritional values:

Energy: 716 g, Protein: 28 g, Carbohydrates: 25 g, fibbers: 2 g, Total Fat: 55 g, Sodium: 326 mg, Phosphorus: 215 mg, Potassium: 340 mg

166. Protein-free spaghetti with clams

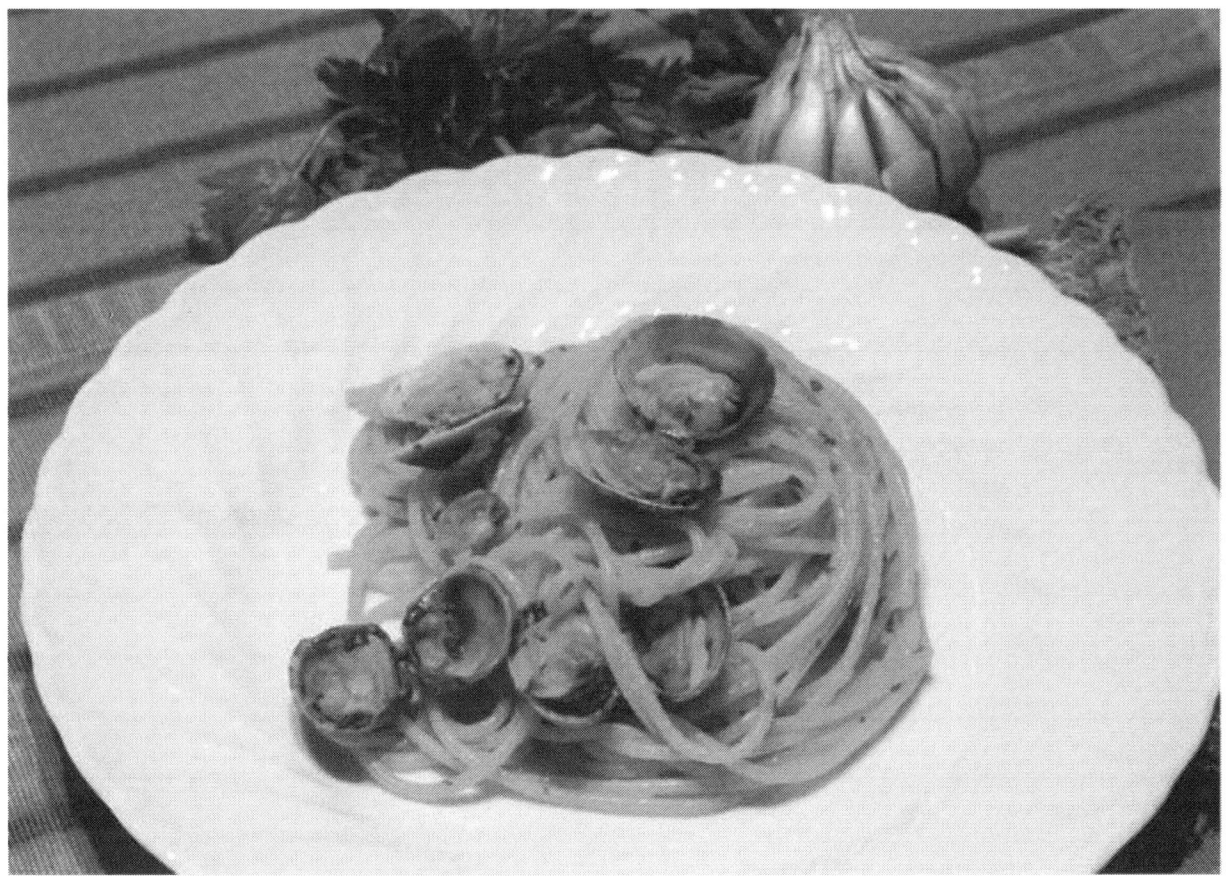

Serving: 1 - 4

Ingredients:

- 300 g of protein-free spaghetti
- A pinch of coarse salt for the pasta water
- 1 kg of clams (about 100 gr without the shell)
- 1 clove of garlic
- 10 g of chopped parsley
- 2 tablespoons of oil
- A grind of pepper

Preparation:

1. Soak the clams in water and coarse salt for about 1 hour to clean them of any impurities, then drain and wash them several times with fresh water, moving them a lot with your hands to make sure they lose all the sand they have inside.
2. In a large pan, fry the finely chopped garlic (or simply crushed if you want to remove it later), add the clams and let them open over high heat. Once opened, remove from the heat, remove

some shells and filter the liquid released during cooking. Clams are usually tasty and you don't need to add salt.

3. In the meantime, you will have boiled the water for the spaghetti, which you will cook very al dente and which you will pass, with the special spaghetti ladle, directly from the water of the pot to the pan with the clams and their liquid to complete the cooking without being too "dry". Add the parsley and, if you like it, a sprinkle of pepper.

The use of protein-free paste must be prescribed by the nephrologist. The soaking and washing of the clams must be added to the preparation time.

Nutritional values:

Protein: 3 g, Calories: 318 kcal, Low potassium 2 *, Low Phosphorus, Lipids: 6 g, Cholesterol: 13 mg

167. Salmon with horseradish cream

Serving: 2

Ingredients:

Sauce

- ¾ cup low-fat sour cream
- ¼ cup mayonnaise
- 2 Tbsp. grated horseradish
- 2 tbsp. chopped fresh basil
- 1 tbsp. fresh lemon juice
- 1 tbsp. soy sauce

Salmon

- 3 tbsp. tablespoon vegetable oil
- 1 tbsp. tablespoon soy sauce
- 1 small clove of garlic, minced
- ¼ tsp. black pepper
- 6 x 6 oz (170 g) salmon fillet
- Vegetable oil spray

Preparation:

Sauce:

- Combine all ingredients in a small bowl. Cover and refrigerate until use.

Salmon:

- Beat together oil, soy sauce, garlic, and pepper in a small bowl. Coat the salmon fillets with the mixture. Cook the fillets on a grill or in a skillet until the centre becomes opaque, about 4 minutes per side. Arrange the salmon on a plate and serve with a tsp. of sauce.

Nutritional values:

Power: 278 g, Protein: 24 g, Carbohydrates: 5.4 g, Total Fat: 17.6 g, Sodium: 376 mg, Potassium: 460 mg, Phosphorus: 302 mg

168. Sole rolls

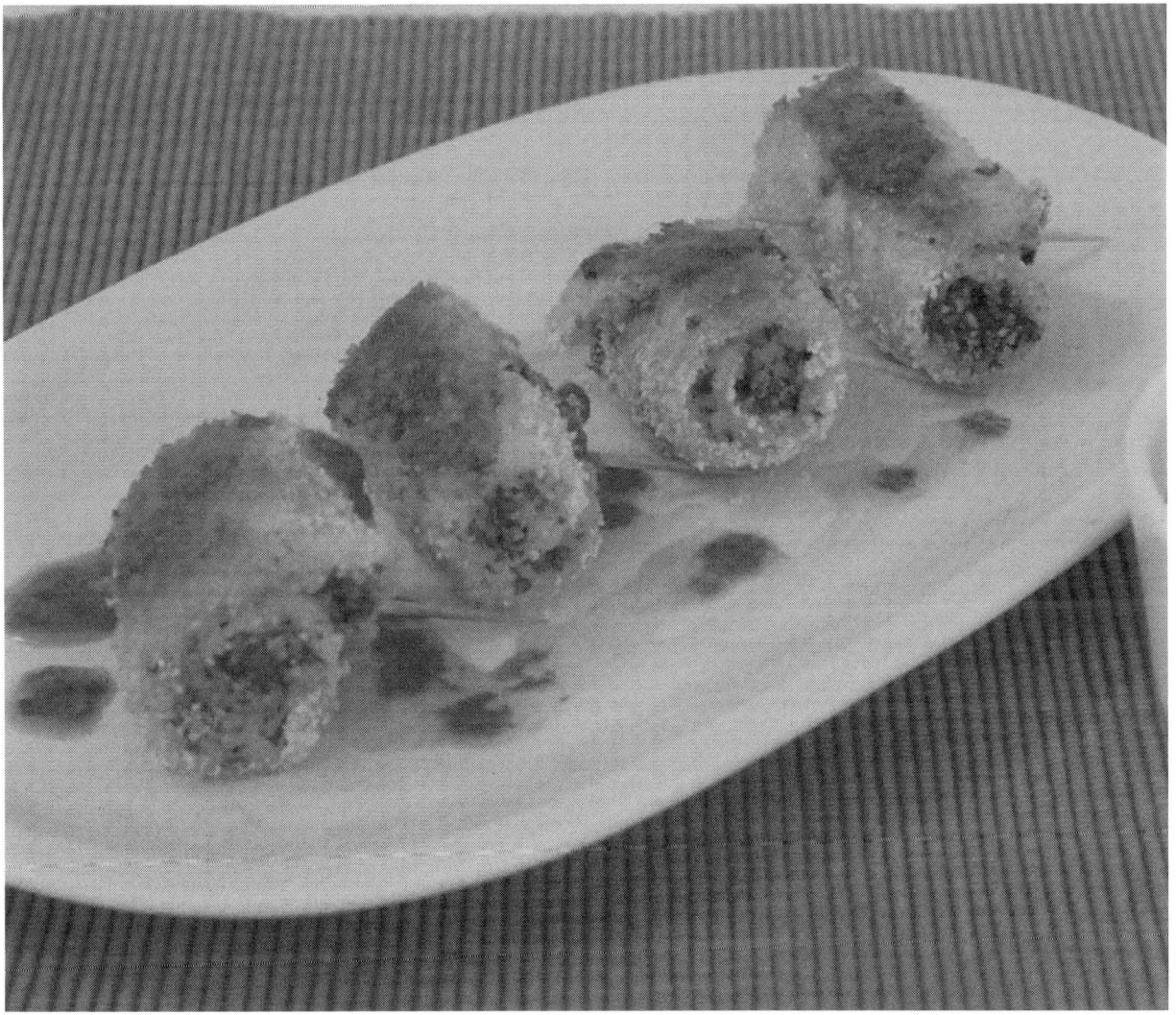

Servings: 1 - 2

Ingredients:

- 200 g of sole fillets (6 rolls)
- 15 g of capers in brine

- 1 clove of garlic
- A sprig of parsley
- 25 g of breadcrumbs
- A grind of pepper
- A pinch of salt
- 10 g of extra virgin olive oil

FOR THE SAUCE

- 1 lemon
- A sprig of parsley
- A sprig of fresh oregano
- 1 small clove of garlic
- 20 g of oil
- Salt and pepper

Preparation:

1. Chop the parsley with the garlic and capers and add the mince to the breadcrumbs. Season with a tablespoon of oil and a sprinkle of pepper to form the mixture that will serve as a filling for the rolls.
2. Spread the fillets of sole on the baking sheet covered with parchment paper, salt them lightly, sprinkle them with the stuffing and close them into rolls, stopping them with a toothpick. Lightly bread them and grease them with a little oil. Bake at 200 ° for about 10-15 '.
3. For the sauce, finely chop the garlic and parsley with the oregano leaves, add a little salt and a grind of pepper, lemon juice, and oil. Emulsify so that the oil and lemon blend into a single liquid and let it rest out of the fridge.
4. Serve the rolls hot seasoned with the sauce.

I chose sole for our rolls because it is a lean fish, easily digestible, and is among the fish with the lowest phosphorus content. To try!

Nutritional values:

Protein: 18 g, Calories: 261 kcal, Potassium 7 *, Medium Phosphorus, Lipids: 17 g, Cholesterol: 25 mg

169. Swordfish rolls with mango sauce

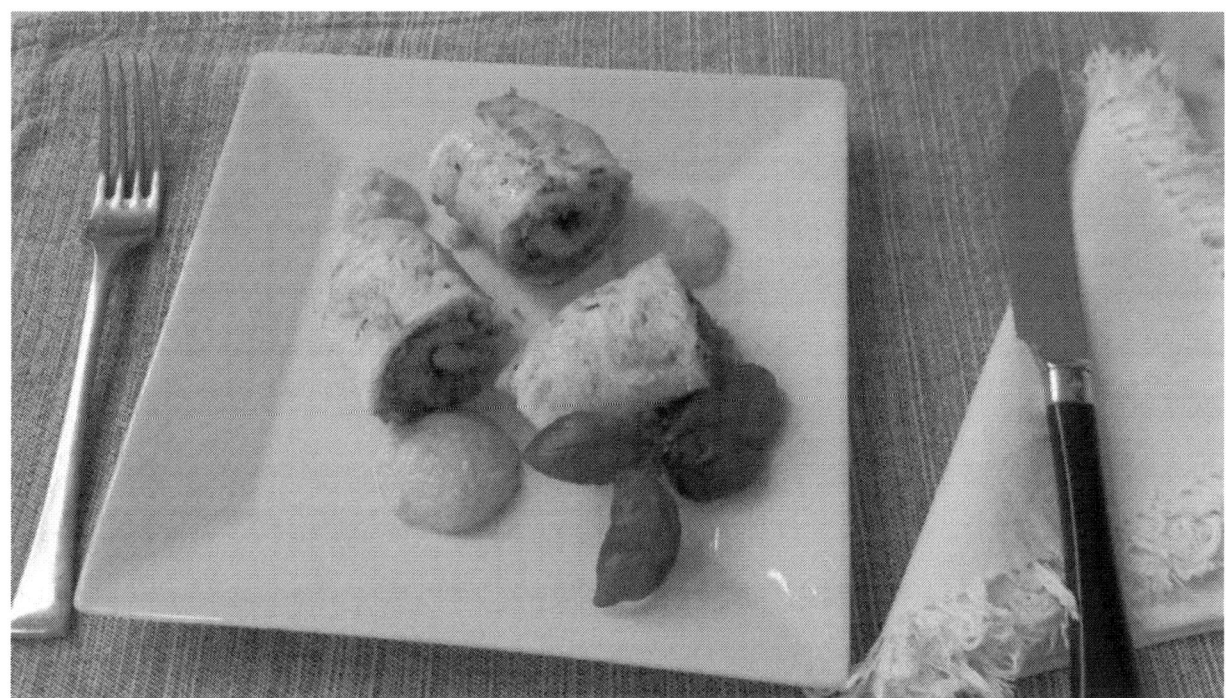

Serving: 1

Ingredients:

- 8 slices of swordfish, 480 g
- Crumb of homemade bread 100 g
- Zest of 1 lemon
- A sprig of basil
- 10 g of extra virgin olive oil
- A pinch of salt
- A grind of pepper

FOR THE MANGO SAUCE

- 1 ripe mango, about 500 g
- Fresh ginger, already peeled, 30 g
- Extra virgin olive oil 10 g
- A pinch of salt
- A grind of pepper

Preparation:

1. First, prepare the mango sauce: take a ripe mango, remove the peel with a smooth blade knife, and cut the pulp into coarse pieces. Also, peel the ginger and grate it inside a tall and narrow

container, then add the mango, season with extra virgin olive oil, a pinch of salt and pepper and blend with a hand blender until you get a creamy sauce and homogeneous.
2. Now prepare the filling of the rolls: cut the crumb of fresh bread into cubes and put it in a blender, then add the washed and dried basil leaves (keep the smaller ones aside for the final garnish), the grated zest of a lemon, extra virgin olive oil, salt and pepper and blend until you get quite fine and uniform crumbs.
3. Take the slices of swordfish and add a spoonful of the mixture thus obtained, distributing it evenly over the entire surface, taking care to leave the edges free. Fold the longer sides inwards, then roll the slice on itself from bottom to top and continue like this to form all the rolls. Heat a non-stick pan with a drizzle of oil, place the rolls with the closure down and cook over medium-high heat for about a minute so that it seals well, then turn them slowly until all sides they will have taken a uniform colour: in all, it will take 2-3 minutes. Transfer the cooked rolls to a serving dish using kitchen tongs so as not to pierce them, add a few drops of mango sauce and the basil leaves that you had kept aside.
4. We recommend consuming the swordfish rolls at the moment. Mango sauce can be frozen.
5. For the mango sauce, it is recommended to use olive oil with a delicate flavour, otherwise you can replace it with the same amount of seed oil.

Nutritional values:

Protein: 21.3 g, Calories: 275 kcal, Potassium 11 *, High Phosphorus, Lipids: 11 g, Cholesterol: 84 mg

170. White mussel soup

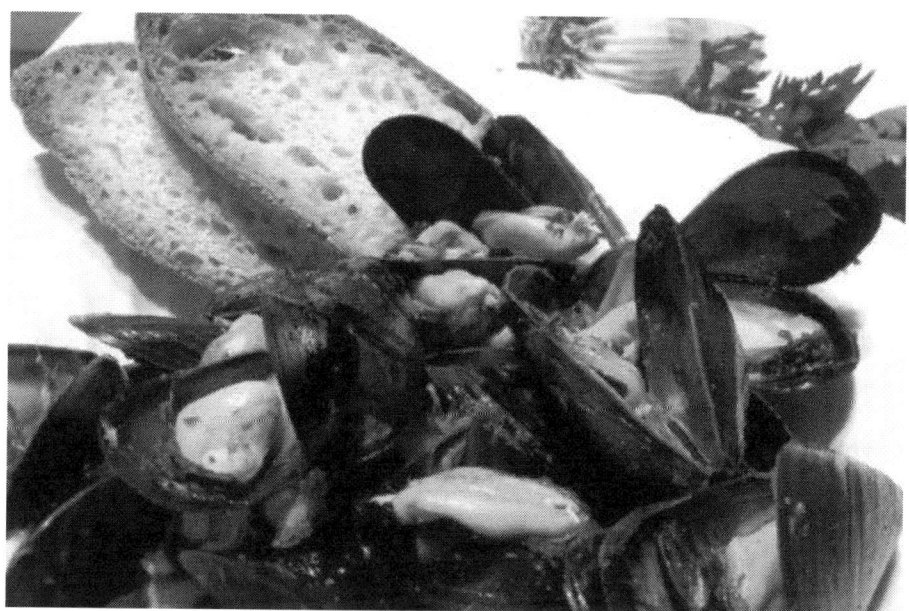

Servings: 1 - 4

Ingredients:

- 1 kg of mussels
- A sprig of parsley
- 2 cloves of garlic
- 20 g of oil
- 4 slices of homemade bread (300 g)
- A pinch of salt
- Black pepper

Preparation:

1. Carefully clean the mussels by removing the "beard" and rubbing them under running water with an aluminium sponge to obtain a perfectly clean surface of the shell.
2. Heat a drizzle of olive oil in a saucepan large enough to hold all the mussels, fry the garlic and add the mussels by letting them open over high heat. A few minutes will be enough.
3. Add the chopped parsley and serve the mussels with their cooking sauce and a slice of toasted homemade bread.

A tomato-free version to reduce potassium!

Nutritional values:

Protein: 12 g, Calories: 202 kcal, Potassium: 7 *, Medium Phosphorus, Lipids: 7 g, Cholesterol: 97 mg

CHAPTER SIXTEEN: Smoothies, Juices and Beverages

171. Seasonal berry drinks

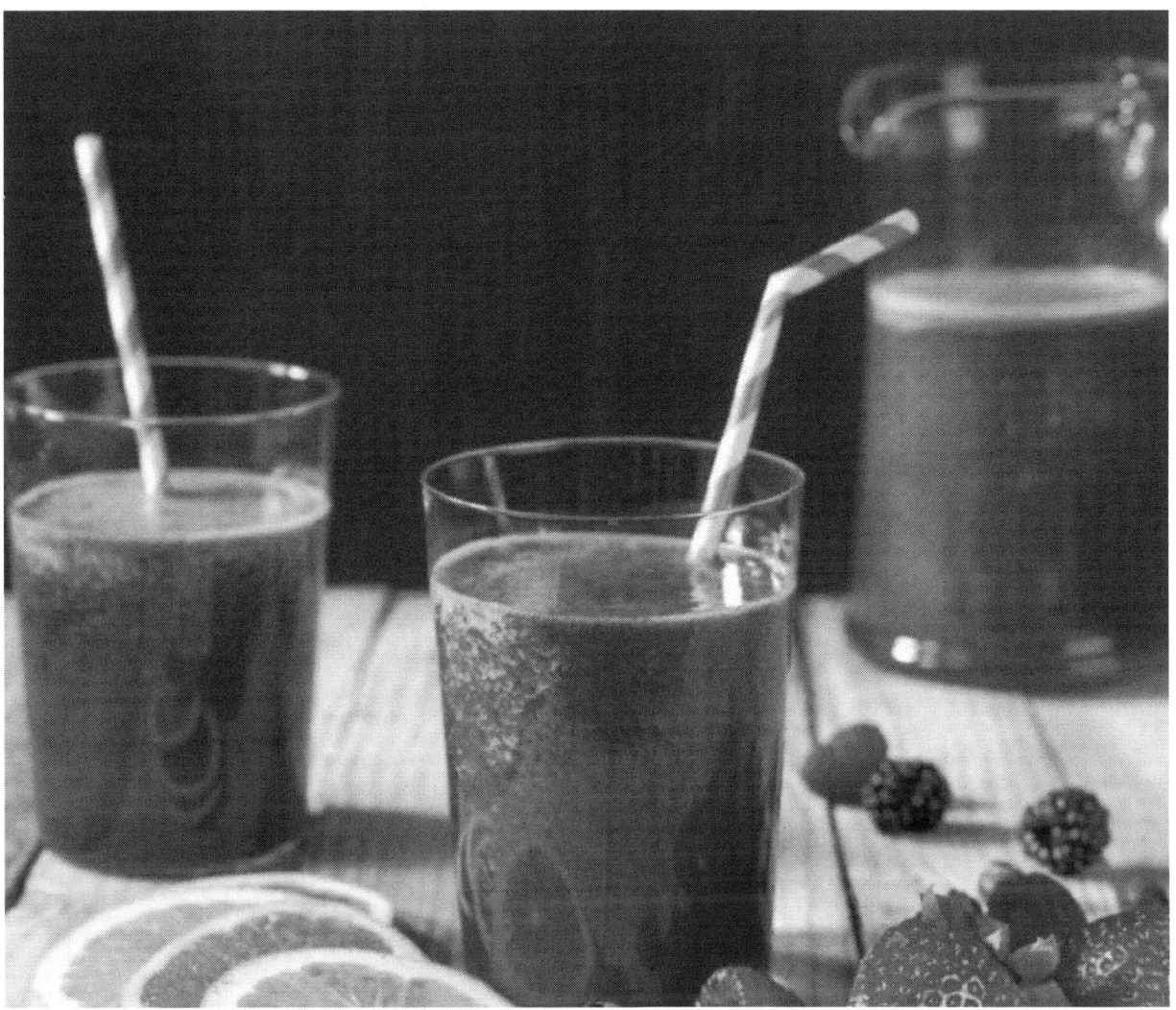

Serving 1

Ingredients:

- 250 mL of water
- 1 C. maple syrup or water
- 1/2 cup of seasonal berries

Preparation:

1. Mash the berries with a fork in a mug.
2. Add water as well as syrup or maple water.
3. Mix and enjoy.

Nutritional values:

Energy: 67.4 g, Proteins: 0.3 g, Carbohydrates: 17.1 g, fibbers: 1 g, Total Fat: .2 g, Sodium: 5.2 mg, Phosphorus: 12.55 mg, Potassium: 119.26 mg

172. Fresh Lemonade

Ingredients:

- Two lemons
- 8 cups water

Preparation:

Squeeze two lemons (1/2 cup lemon juice), into 8 cups of water. You can use a regular juicer, or you can buy pre-squeezed lemon juice. Serve with ice cubes and a hint of mint for flavour. Drink throughout the day. You can add sugar or a sugar substitute if desired, but try to limit your sugar levels to reduce your risk of kidney stones. For more information on kidney stones see our fact sheet.

Nutritional values:

Energy: 4 g, Proteins: 0.1 g, Carbohydrates: 1.4 g, Sodium: 10 mg, Phosphorus: 1.0 mg, Potassium: 20 mg

173. Blueberry Shake

Ingredients:

- 1 ¼ cup pineapple juice
- 2 cups frozen blueberries (lightly thawed)
- ¾ cup pasteurized egg whites
- 2 tbsp. sugar or Splenda
- ½ cup water (a little more or a little less depending on the consistency desired)

Preparation:

Put all the ingredients in a blender and puree. Enjoy your meal!

Nutritional values:

Energy: 155.4 g, Proteins: 7.4 g, Carbohydrates: 31.1 g, fibbers: 3 g, Total Fat: 0.75 g, Sodium: 104.1 mg, Phosphorus: 27.5 mg, Potassium: 289.4 mg

CHAPTER SEVENTEEN: Low-Protein Desserts

174. Low-Protein Apple Pie

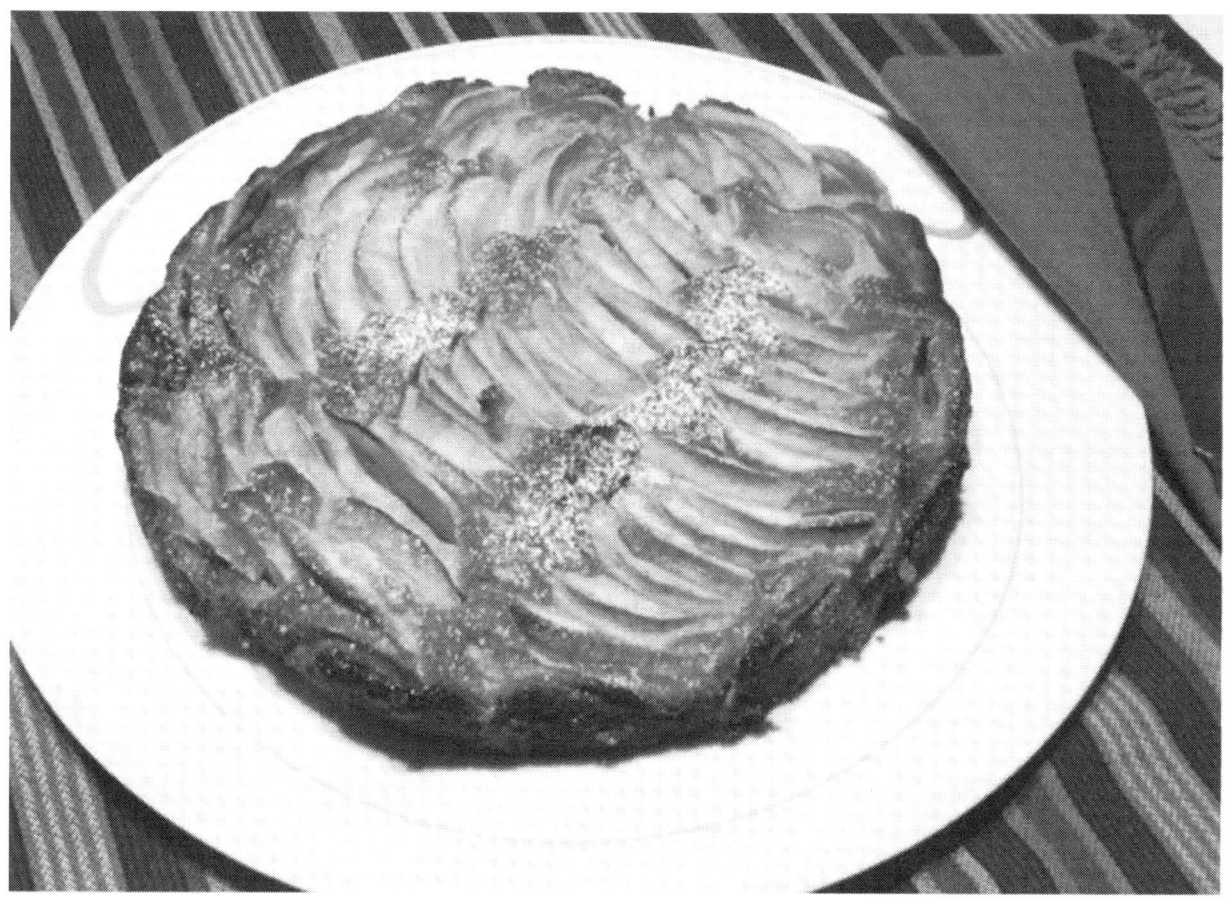

Servings: 1 - 8

Ingredients:

- 2 large rennet apples (about 500 gr)
- Low-protein flour 125 gr
- Sugar 100 gr
- Brown sugar 1 tbsp
- Butter 100 gr
- 2 whole eggs
- Low-protein milk 30 ml
- Grated lemon zest (or, to taste, freshly grated ginger)
- 1 teaspoon of baking powder
- A pinch of salt

- (TO COMPLETE) Powdered sugar to taste

Preparation:

1. Whip the butter, previously softened out of the refrigerator, with the sugar, salt, and lemon peel (or fresh grated ginger) with the electric whisk (or in the robot), until they become fluffy. Then add the eggs, one at a time, continuing to whip at high speed. Do not add the second egg if the first has not been well absorbed and whipped, making the dough fluffy. Then, lowering the speed, add the flour with the yeast and the milk.
2. Mix all the ingredients well and pour the mixture into a pan (diameter 25 cm) previously greased and floured; at this point, arrange the apple slices in the mixture, which you will have cut at the moment so as not to blacken them, sprinkle with a little brown sugar and a few flakes of butter and bake in a preheated oven at 180 ° for 40-45 minutes.
3. Let it cool and sprinkle with a little icing sugar.

The low-protein version of apple pie is to be used when the nephrologist prescribes the use of protein-free products. The use of protein-free flour and milk doesn't involve particular recommendations.

Nutritional values:

Protein: 2 g, Calories: 252 kcal, Low potassium: 2 *, Minimum phosphorus, Lipids: 12 g, Cholesterol: 87 mg

175. Low-Protein Carrot Cake

Servings: 1 - 10

Ingredients:

- 200 gr of grated carrots
- 180 gr of protein-free flour
- 100 grams of sugar
- 50 gr of butter
- 2 eggs
- 50 gr of soaked raisins (in marsala or cognac)
- 40 gr of walnut kernels
- 8 gr of yeast
- 6 small macaroons (about 20 g)
- (TO COMPLETE) Powdered sugar to taste

Preparation:

1. Grease a plum cake pan with a little butter and sprinkle it with the crumbled amaretti biscuits. Grate the carrots. Blend the walnuts with part of the sugar.
2. In a large bowl, whisk the egg yolks with the remaining sugar, gradually adding the softened butter, the walnuts blended with the sugar, the well-squeezed raisins, the flour with the baking powder, the carrots, and finally incorporated the whipped egg whites.
3. Bake at 180 degrees for about 45 minutes.

The use of protein-free flour and milk does not involve particular recommendations. I always remember that the use of protein-free products must be prescribed by the nephrologist.

Nutritional values:

Protein: 3 g, Calories: 211 kcal, Potassium: 3 *, Low Phosphorus, Lipids: 8 g, Cholesterol 57 mg

176. Low-Protein Apple Strudel

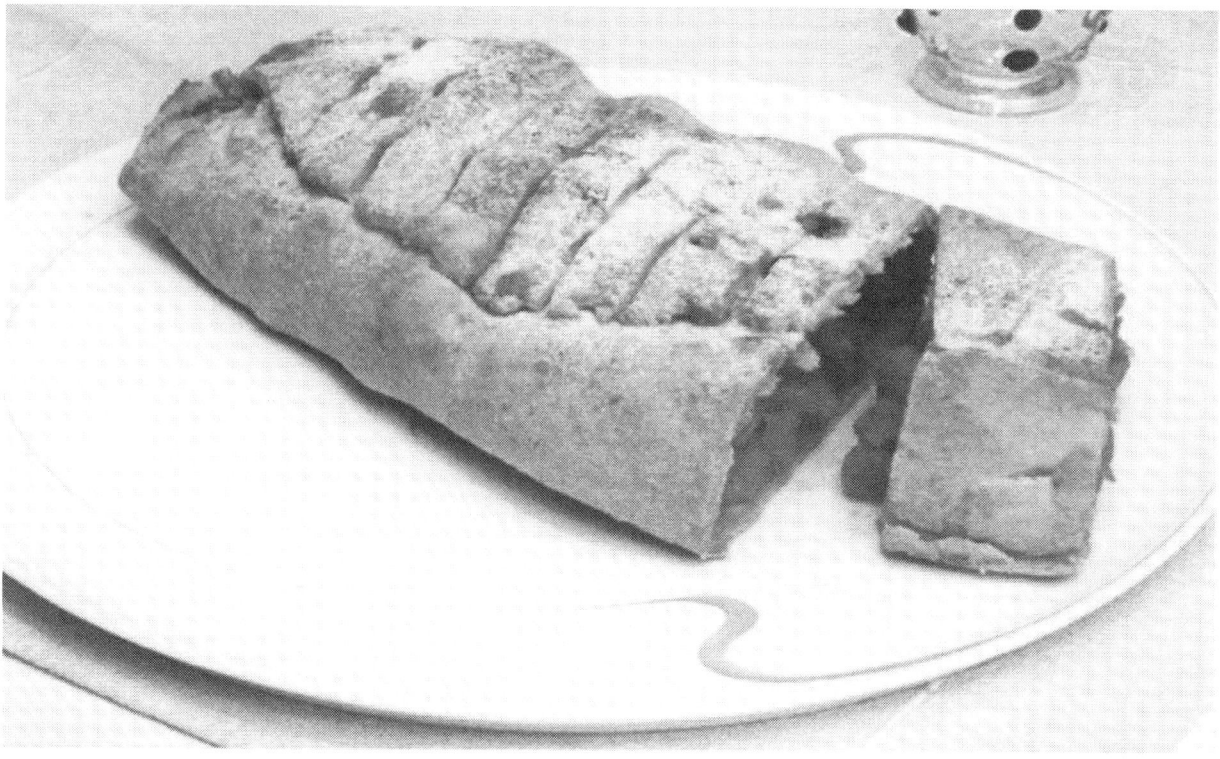

Servings: 1 - 8

Ingredients:

FOR THE PASTA

- 250 grams of protein-free flour
- 1 whole egg

- 50 gr of melted butter
- 50 ml of water

FOR THE STUFFING

- 700 gr of Renette apples (4 apples)
- 100 grams of brown sugar
- 85 grams of raisins
- 10 walnut kernels (45 g)
- 50 gr of melted butter
- Cinnamon to taste
- (TO COMPLETE) Powdered sugar to taste

Preparation:

1. Mix the flour with the egg and warm water and then add the melted butter.
2. When the dough is smooth and soft, form a ball, wrap it in plastic wrap and place it in the refrigerator for about 30 minutes.
3. For the filling: peel the apples and cut them into slices. In a large bowl, mix the apples with the other filling ingredients.
4. Roll out the dough to form a rectangle of about 30 x 40 cm, brush with some of the melted butter, and place the apple mixture in the centre.
5. Close by matching the edges so that the mixture does not come out during cooking. Brush with the remaining melted butter and score the surface with oblique cuts.
6. Bake for 45 minutes at 180 degrees.
7. Before serving, sprinkle with icing sugar.

The version with protein-free products must be prescribed by the nephrologist.

Nutritional values:

Protein: 3 g, Calories: 368 kcal, Potassium: 5 *, Low Phosphorus, Lipids: 15 g, Cholesterol 59 mg

177. Low-Protein Panna Cotta with Strawberries and Raspberries

Serving: for one low protein portion (with low protein milk)

Ingredients:

- 500 ml of fresh cream
- 500 ml of low-protein milk
- 160 grams of sugar
- 1 vanilla bean
- 8 sheets of isinglass or 4 sachets of Agar equal to 8 gr

- (FOR THE GASKET)
- 500 gr of strawberries
- 130 gr of raspberries
- 20 grams of sugar
- The juice of ½ lemon

Preparation:

1. Pour the cream and milk with the sugar into a saucepan. Add the vanilla bean, which you will have divided into two parts with a knife lengthwise, and leave it to infuse while they heat up to a boil, then remove it while the seeds will remain in the liquid.
2. When the liquids are hot, before boiling, add the agar-agar and let it boil, stirring constantly for at least a couple of minutes. If, on the other hand, you use isinglass let the cream and milk cool before adding it, after having softened it in cold water and squeezed it well.
3. At this point, distribute the panna cotta in the glasses and place it in the refrigerator for at least 3 hours before garnishing.
4. For the garnish, carefully wash the strawberries and raspberries, slice the strawberries and distribute them in the glasses with a few raspberries. Separately, prepare a sauce with a part of the strawberries (about 100 g out of the 500 total) 20 g of sugar, and lemon juice: blend everything and pour a spoonful into each glass.

In this case, the reduction of proteins is obtained with the use of protein-free milk.

Nutritional values:

Protein: 2 g, Calories: 195 kcal, Potassium: 3 *, Minimum phosphorus, Lipids: 10 g, Cholesterol: 33 mg

178. Low-Protein Tart with Citrus Jam

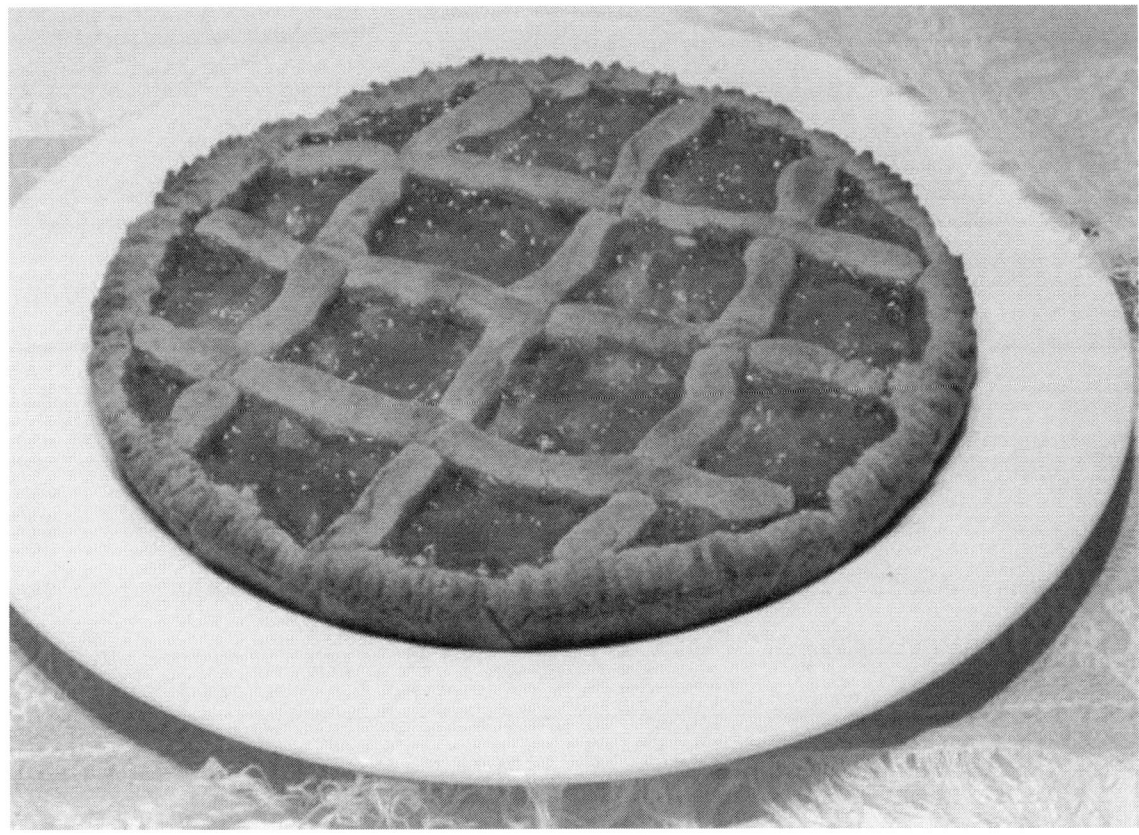

Servings: 1 - 8

Ingredients:

- 500 Low-protein flour 200 g
- Butter 100 gr
- Sugar 100 gr
- 1 modest pinch of salt
- 2 egg yolks
- Grated lemon peel
- Mixed citrus marmalade 300 gr (oranges, lemons, grapefruit)

Preparation:

1. Prepare the shortcrust pastry by placing the sifted flour on a pastry board, in the centre put the butter into small pieces, sugar, salt, egg yolks, and grated lemon zest (preferably using an untreated lemon, which must still be well washed and dried).
2. Knead all the ingredients with your hands and form a ball that you will rest in the refrigerator for at least half an hour, covered with a cloth or wrapped in parchment paper that you will later

use to cover the baking pan. If you have a food processor you can knead everything and only at the end complete the dough by hand forming a ball.
3. Once removed from the refrigerator, divide the dough keeping a small part of it for the strips of garnish, and spread the thickest part in a cake pan (diameter 25 cm.), Previously covered with parchment paper, cover with the jam, which you will carefully smooth a spatula, and with the leftover mixture provide strips that you will arrange in the shape of a grid on the mixture.
4. Bake at 180 degrees for about 30-40 minutes. Let it cool before turning it out into the serving dish.

The low-protein version is for the event that the nephrologist prescribes a reduction of proteins in the diet. The use of protein-free flour will make the dough more "floury" but it will compact easily after the first manipulations.

Nutritional values:

Protein: 1 g, Calories: 342 kcal, Low Potassium, Minimum Phosphorus, Lipids: 12 g, Cholesterol: 90 mg

CONCLUSION

Composition of Some Types of Vegetables and Fruits

I want to report the composition of some types of vegetables and fruit. The data refer to 100 g of raw product.

VEGETABLES	Calories	Proteins	Lipids	Glycides	Calcium	Sodium	Potassium	Phosphorous
	Kcal	g	g	g	mg	mg	mg	mg
Artichokes	46.9	3.3	0.2	2.1	43.7	93.7	370.3	89.8
Asparagus	22.4	2.2	0.1	2.1	1.9	1.5	273.1	56.7
White bean	336.1	21.1	1.2	5.5	173.1	12	1541.7	445.4
Broccoli	27.3	2.9	0.5	2	47.7	27.3	325	65.9
Cabbage	24.3	5.4	0.3	2.6	47.1	18.6	245.7	22.8
Carrot	43.7	1.1	0.2	6.6	26.6	34.4	323.4	43.7
Cauliflower	24	2	0.2	2.4	22	30	304	44
Aubergine	26.8	1	0.2	3.4	7.3	2.4	217	21.9
Fennel	31.8	1.1	0.2	0.2	50	52.3	413.6	50
Leek	61.4	1.6	0.2	3.9	59.1	20.5	179.5	34.1
Yellow peppers	27.2	1	0.2	2.5	11.1	0.3	212.2	23.9
Pumpkin	25.9	1	0.2	4.5	20.7	1.7	339.7	44.8
Radicchio	25	1.5	0.5		20	20	300	40
Spinach	23.3	3	0.3	0.3	100	80	556.7	50
Zucchini	13.8	1.2	0.1	1.7	15.4	3.1	247.7	32.3
Potatoes	63.5	2.3	0.6	0.1	4.7	3.5	515.3	
Tomatoes	21.1	4.7	0.3	2.7	4.4	8.9	222.2	24.4
Green beans	30.9	1.8	0.2	2.5	36.4	5.5	209.1	38.2

FRUITS	Calories	Proteins	Lipids	Glycides	Calcium	Sodium	Potassium	Phosphorous
	Kcal	g	g	g	mg	mg	mg	mg
Apples	42.7	0.3	0	10.5	2.9	2.2	74.6	
Apricots	47.6	1.3	0.2	5.1	8	0.7	176.1	11.6
Bananas	92	1.1	0.3	18.5	5.3	0.7	396	20
Cherries	72.2	1.3	1	14.3	15.3	0	223.6	19.4
Blueberries	50	0.4	0.2	8.5	6.3	0	70.8	8.3
Currants	55.3	1.4	0.2	9.5	32.1	1.8	275	44.6
Figs	74	0.8	0.4	15.8	36	0	232	14
Kiwi	67.6	1.3	0.7	10.8	40.5		324.3	
Mango	65.2	0.5	0.3	14.8	28.4	1.9	156	11.1
Melon	37.3	0.7	0	8.2	14.9	18.7	208.9	
Orange	40	1.3	0.3	5.8	70.1	2.3	196.5	22.3
Peaches	42.9	0.7	8.7	0.1	5.1	0	196.9	12.2
Pears	58.5	0.4	0.4	10.5	11	0	124.4	11
Khaki	128	0.8	0.4	32	28	0	312	24
Pineapple	48.7	0.4	0.4	11.1	6.4	1.3	112.8	6.4
Dried plum	271.4	2.9	0.4	32.9	17.9	10.7	725	
Strawberry	30.1	0.6	0.4	4.7	14.5	1.2	166.3	19.3

These data were extrapolated from the text "Nutrients in food" by Elizabeth S. Hands published by Lippincott Williams & Wilkins.

What the Numbers Associated with the Most Common Diets Want to Say

The number associated with diets (e.g., 0.8g / kg/day) indicates the amount of protein there is in the diet, related to the weight of the person.

Total protein, allowed by the diet, is calculated by multiplying the number by the weight of the person.

Weight x number associated with the diet = total protein

Examples:

A) a diet of 0.6 g / kg/day for a person who weighs 70 kg, means that daily this person must introduce an amount of protein equal to:

70 x 0.6 = 42 g / kg / day

B) a diet 0.8 g / kg / day for a person weighing 70 kg, means that daily this person must introduce an amount of protein equal to:

70 x 0.8 = 56 g / kg / day

A Practical Strategy to Reduce the Potassium Content in Vegetables

To reduce the potassium content in vegetables, you can cook them as follows:

- ✓ Remove the peel and outer leaves of the vegetables if possible.
- ✓ Cut into small cubes to create a larger contact surface between the vegetable and the cooking water.
- ✓ Wash the cut vegetables under running water, immerse them in plenty of unsalted water and leave them to soak for 20-30 minutes.
- ✓ Put the vegetables to cook in plenty of unsalted water. After few minutes from boiling with new unsalted water until cooked.
- ✓ Drain everything and season with oil.

The cooking water cannot be used either as broth or as a cooking liquid. If you salt the cooking water of the vegetables, the osmotic effect is reduced and therefore the passage of ions (sodium, potassium, etc.) from food to water.

And this is the end.

I wish you good luck in your battle, even if I already know for sure that these recipes will make a big difference, as they did for a person dear to me, giving us smiles even in the least happy moments and above all hope!

Dorothy Vandekamp.

Printed in Great Britain
by Amazon